Neonatal Care

A Textbook for Student Midwives and Nurses

Edited by Amanda Williamson and Kenda Crozier

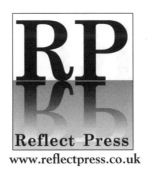

Reflect Press

www.reflectpress.co.uk

First published in 2008

ISBN: 978 1 906052 09 6

British Library Cataloguing in Publication Data
A catalogue record for this book is available from the British Library

The authors and publisher have made every attempt to ensure the content of this book is up to date and accurate. However, health care knowledge and information is changing all the time so the reader is advised to double-check any information in this text on drug usage, treatment procedures, the use of equipment, etc. to confirm that it complies with the latest safety recommendations, standards of practice and legislation, as well as local Trust policies and procedures. Students are advised to check with their tutor and/or mentor before carrying out the procedures in this textbook.

Production project management by Deer Park Productions

Typeset by PDQ Typesetting

Cover design by Oxmed

Printed and bound by Bell& Bain Ltd, Glasgow

Distributed by BEBC, Albion Close, Parkstone, Poole, Dorset BH12 3LL

Published by Reflect Press Ltd
11 Attwyll Avenue
Exeter
Devon, EX2 5HN
UK
01392 204400

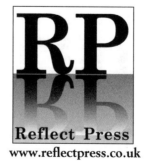

Reflect Press
www.reflectpress.co.uk

Neonatal C

A Textbook for Student Midwives and Nurses

Contents

Preface

The aim of this book is to provide student midwives, student nurses, nursery nurses and senior health care assistants with a practical and theoretical guide to all aspects of basic neonatal care.

The book has a gradual progression that leads the reader through the types of neonatal services available and the care the neonate may require and why. The midwife or nurse's role in facilitating neonatal care within the family is also explored and explained. Consideration is given to cultural and diversity issues as well as legal and professional matters pertinent to caring for the neonate.

All chapters are mapped, where appropriate, to the NHS Knowledge and Skills Framework (2004) and the Nursing and Midwifery Council (NMC) Standards of Proficiency for pre-registration midwifery education (2004), allowing clear identification of the relevance of each chapter to these. In doing so, we have made use of relevant expertise from the fields of education and clinical practice.

List of contributors

Amanda Williamson is a neonatal/midwifery lecturer at the University of East Anglia and former Lead for Clinical Standards on the Neonatal Intensive Care Unit at the Norfolk and Norwich University NHS Hospital Trust. Her interests in teaching include neonatal care as well as legal and professional issues. She teaches on the pre-registration midwifery courses as well as being unit leader for the Neonatal (Intensive Care) Nursing Unit, Enhanced Neonatal Nursing Practice Unit, Neuro-Behavioural Physiological Assessment of Newborn Unit and unit leader for the MSc Advanced Practitioner – Neonatal Course.

Kenda Crozier is a lecturer in midwifery at the School of Nursing and Midwifery, University of East Anglia. She is currently the Lead for the MSc Advanced Practitioner programme midwifery pathway. Her teaching experience includes pre- and post-registration and postgraduate teaching and supervision in the areas of midwifery and neonatal care. Her special interests include the development of competence and the use of technology in supporting care.

Mary Melley is Lead Nurse, Tyrone County Hospital, Northern Ireland and part-time Neonatal Sister, Erne Hospital. She is also a Supervisor of Midwives. Her professional interests include critical care decisions in fetal and neonatal medicine; the impact of antenatal screening on neonatal survival and disability and neonatal sepsis.

Cathy Coppinger has worked as a midwife in hospital, community and integrated team settings. She has been a Head of Midwifery, Regional Child Health Co-ordinator for the East of England and more recently Quality and Audit Development Co-ordinator at the Royal College of Midwives. Cathy completed the Examination of the Newborn unit at the University of East Anglia in 2005. She is currently employed as a Programme Manager at the UK Newborn Screening Centre, based at Great Ormond Street Hospital.

Karen Hill is currently employed as a practice development midwife at Queen Elizabeth Hospital, Kings Lynn and has completed the Examination of the Newborn unit. She was formerly the practice facilitator for the pre-registration midwifery course at the University of East Anglia.

Karen Bates is lecturer in midwifery at the University of East Anglia and a Supervisor of Midwives. She is currently course director for the post-registration midwifery programmes and has a special interest in professional communication.

Julie Mullett is a qualified midwife and Advanced Neonatal Nurse Practitioner who has been working with neonates for 15 years. She is currently an Operational Manager at the Norfolk and Norwich University NHS Hospital Trust.

Nicki Young is a lecturer in midwifery at the University of East Anglia. As a qualified midwife she was a member of the Princess Mary's Royal Air Force Nursing Service and has worked as a nurse and midwife in Canada and Saudi Arabia. Currently she is studying for a Doctorate in Education at the Centre for Applied Research in Education at the University of East Anglia. Her research interests include clinical decision-making in midwifery, the midwifery care received by women who undergo termination of pregnancy for fetal abnormality, and the midwifery management of childbearing emergencies.

Charlene Lobo is a health visitor by profession. She currently works as a lecturer in Primary Care and Public Health at the University of East Anglia and has a special interest in developing practice in safeguarding children.

Chapter 1

Introduction to the Neonate and Neonatal Services

Amanda Williamson

Chapter aims

To explore the context of neonatal care and the services available to care for the neonate.

Learning outcomes

At the end of this chapter you will be able to:

- understand the definitions of babies and the importance of this in planning appropriate neonatal care;
- discuss the categories of neonatal care;
- articulate the differences between the types of care level (3, 2 and 1) neonatal units may offer;
- demonstrate an understanding of the role of managed neonatal clinical networks and the impact of National Service Frameworks on neonatal care provision.

Mapping to Standards of Proficiency

Standards of Proficiency for Pre-registration Midwifery Education (SPME)
Works collaboratively with other practitioners and agencies in ways which:

- value their contribution to health and care;
- enable them to participate effectively in the care of women, babies and their families;
- acknowledge the nature of their work and the context in which it is placed.

NHS Knowledge and Skills Framework (NHS KSF)
Core 5, Level 2
e) Uses and maintains resources efficiently and effectively and encourages others to do so.

Standards of Proficiency for Pre-registration Nursing Education
Provide a rationale for nursing care delivered which takes account of social, cultural, spiritual, legal, political and economic influences.

Consult other health care professionals when individual or group needs fall outside the scope of nursing practice.
Establish priorities for care based on individual or group needs.

INTRODUCTION

A neonate may be defined as an infant in the first four weeks of life. For the purposes of this book, instead of neonate the term 'baby' will be used throughout the text.

The main emphasis of this textbook is to examine the role of the health care practitioner in caring for the normal-term baby. However, it is important that you are able to understand the differences between various definitions of babies, such as 'premature' or 'small for gestational age', as identifying babies within these parameters may affect the planning of care to be given.

Length of pregnancy and date of delivery

Gestational weeks in pregnancy are calculated from the date of the first day of the mother's last menstrual period. The relationship between the baby's weight and gestational age is crucial in determining the type of care a baby will receive. The calculated delivery date is formulated by adding nine calendar months and seven days to the date of the first day of the woman's last menstrual period. The duration of pregnancy is based upon Naegele's rule that presumes the duration of pregnancy to be 280 days (Viccars, 2003). With the growing use of ultrasound most women in the United Kingdom are offered an early dating ultrasound scan which will provide a more accurate assessment of gestational age and expected date of delivery. You may see this written as the 'EDD'.

The classification of babies

A 'term' baby is a baby born after 37 completed weeks of pregnancy and before 41 completed weeks of pregnancy. A 'post-term' baby is a baby born after 41 completed weeks of pregnancy (Johnston *et al.*, 2004).

Classification by prematurity

- A premature baby is a baby born before 37 completed weeks of pregnancy (England, 2003).
- A moderately premature baby is a baby born between 35–37 weeks of pregnancy (BLISS, 2004).

- A very premature baby is a baby born between 29–34 weeks of pregnancy (BLISS, 2004).
- An extremely premature baby is a baby born between 24–28 weeks of pregnancy (BLISS, 2004).

Classification by weight

Growth charts may be used to assess if the baby is an appropriate weight for its gestational age. However, genetic and environmental factors should also be taken into consideration when assessing if a baby is an appropriate weight for its gestational age. Centile charts are often used to plot a baby's weight (see below).

- A low birth weight (LBW) baby is a baby who weighs 2 500 g or less at birth.
- A very low birth weight baby (VLBW) is a baby who weighs below 1 500 g at birth.
- An extremely low birth weight baby (ELBW) is a baby who weighs below 1 000 g at birth.

(Papageorgiou and Bardin, 1999)

> **Information box 1**
>
> Centile charts are often used to plot a baby's growth over a period of time. Centile charts only show the weight of the baby within a statistical distribution. This means that they only show how the baby's weight compares with that of other babies. For an example of a centile chart go to **www.patient.co.uk/showdoc/40001849**
>
> Centile charts for a baby's growth are shown as a graph. The 50th centile (middle line) usually represents the average expected weight. This means that if a baby weighs less than average it will be below the 50th centile and if the baby's weight is above the 50th centile it weighs more than average.

Types of low birth weight babies

- Appropriate for Gestational Age (AGA) – these babies are small but their rate of growth is appropriate for their gestation.
- Small for Gestational Age (SGA) – these are babies born at term or later who weigh less than the 10th centile or more than two standard deviations below the mean weight expected for that gestation.
- Small for gestational age and preterm – these are babies who have been born before the 37th completed week of pregnancy and who also weigh

less than the 10th centile or more than two standard deviations below the mean weight expected for that gestation.
- Large for gestational age – these are babies who are considered large for their gestational age because their weight falls over the 90th centile for their gestation.

(England, 2003)

Intrauterine growth restriction

- **Asymmetrical** – asymmetrical growth in a baby (where the head is of a normal size but the body is small) suggests that although body growth has been restricted there has been brain growth.
- **Symmetrical** – symmetrical growth (where the head and body are in proportion) suggests that both brain and body growth have been limited.

(Stables and Rankin, 2005)

The care of these babies will be discussed further in Chapter 8.

WHAT IS NEONATAL CARE?

The importance of good neonatal care must not be underestimated. The care given to women and their babies during pregnancy, childbirth and postnatally can have a significant impact on children's long-term healthy development and their resilience to problems in later life (Department of Health (DH), 2004). Care of the well term baby generally falls under the care of the midwife with support from other health care practitioners. In the Midwives' Rules and Standards it says that the 'midwife is responsible for providing midwifery care ... to a woman and baby during the antenatal, intranatal and postnatal periods' (Nursing and Midwifery Council (NMC), 2004, p. 16). However, other health care professionals, particularly health care assistants or nursery nurses, may be involved in the baby's care during this time.

Currently the duration of community midwifery postnatal care is up to about 10–14 days postnatally and full discharge from maternity services is at six to eight weeks after birth. The *National Service Framework for Children, Young People and Maternity Services* actually recommends that midwifery-led services should provide care to the mother and her baby for at least one month after the birth or from discharge from hospital. They recommend that this could be even longer depending upon individual need (DH, 2004).This is based on a survey undertaken by the National Childbirth Trust which found that women felt they did not have enough on going information and help between 11–30 days after birth compared to up to 10 days after birth (DH, 2004).

In 2006 the National Institute for Health and Clinical Excellence (NICE) published a clinical guideline on routine postnatal care of women and their babies (NICE, 2006). The aim of this guideline is to provide a framework from which a health care professional, in conjunction with parents, can facilitate the health and well-being of a baby up to the age of eight weeks (NICE, 2006). It says that women should 'be offered relevant and timely information to enable them to promote their own and babies' health and well-being and to recognise and respond to problems' (NICE, 2006, p. 6). All health care practitioners caring for babies in the newborn period should be aware of and practise within this guideline. The *National Service Framework for Children, Young People and Maternity Services* says that parents and carers should be given information services and support which will help them to care for their children (DH, 2004). It is important that the health care practitioner is able to offer this service to parents. It is the aim of this book to enable you to achieve this support when caring for babies and their parents.

Categories of neonatal care

There are four categories of neonatal care identified by the British Association of Perinatal Medicine (BAPM, 2001):

- **Normal care** – this is care that is provided for babies who have no medical indication to be in hospital but who remain in hospital because the mother may need support. This could include babies with minor or common medical problems.
- **Special care** – this is care provided for babies who could not reasonably be expected to be looked after at home by their mother. This might include babies who still require naso-gastric tube feeding or who have an unstable temperature. BAPM (2001) recommends that nurses or midwives caring for normal or special care babies should not have responsibility for more than four babies. It is these two categories of babies that will form the main focus of this book.
   The other two categories are:
- **High-dependency care** – this includes babies who are receiving nasal continuous positive airway pressure (NCPAP), who are below 1 000 g (and not fulfilling any intensive care criteria); babies receiving parental nutrition who are having convulsions; babies having oxygen therapy and who are below 1 500 g; babies with neonatal abstinence syndrome, babies requiring specified procedures (but that do not fulfil criteria for intensive care); or babies who require frequent stimulation for apnoeas. These babies should receive care from a nurse who has responsibility for no more than two high-dependency babies (BAPM, 2001).
- **Intensive care** – these are babies with the most complex problems and they should receive one-to-one care by a nurse who also has a post-

registration qualification in neonatal nursing. A competent doctor (in neonatal medicine) should also be available as there is the possibility of sudden deterioration in these babies. This group would include:

- babies who are receiving respiratory support from an endotracheal tube and for 24 hours post extubation;
- babies receiving NCPAP for any part of the day and who are less than five days old;
- babies who are receiving NCPAP and are under 1 000 g for any part of the day and for 24 hours after withdrawal;
- any baby less than 29 weeks' gestation and less than 48 hours old;
- babies requiring major surgery for the pre-operative period and for 24 hours post operatively;
- any baby requiring complex clinical procedures;
- any baby who has a very unstable clinical condition;
- any baby on the day of death.

(BAPM, 2001)

The BAPM (2001) categorised neonatal units into three levels (see Box 2 below).

Information box 2

- Level 1 neonatal units provide special care for babies but do not aim to give continuous high-dependency or intensive care to babies. The units may or may not have medical staff in residence.
- Level 2 neonatal units provide high-dependency neonatal care and could offer some short-term intensive care. The amount of intensive care offered in Level 2 units would be agreed by the neonatal managed clinical networks (NMCN).
- Level 3 neonatal units offer the highest level of care. These neonatal units provide the whole range of neonatal medical care. Not all Level 3 intensive care units will offer specialist services (for example, neonatal surgery). A further unit could be added, that of midwifery level for those babies requiring normal routine care.

(BAPM, 2001)

Transitional care and outreach support

A further type of care that may be given is called 'transitional care'. This care is defined by BLISS (2004, p. 22) as 'special care for babies who are being cared for by their mothers in preparation for going home. Mother and baby share a room and this type of care may involve light therapy for jaundice, tube feeding and intravenous antibiotics'. Generally, the criteria for suitable babies are identified and agreed within the local NHS Trust between neonatologists and maternity services. The criteria usually are that the baby is well, is between 32–36 weeks' gestation and has a weight range of 1.5–2.5 kg (Bromley, 2000). Other babies may be included depending on the NHS Trust's preference. Babies that might be included within the criteria are those who have poor temperature control, infants of diabetic mothers, babies requiring gastric tube feeds or any baby that is medically well but requires a higher level of care than can be given on the postnatal ward. It is generally the responsibility of the midwife on the delivery suite or the postnatal ward to make the referral to transitional care. This means that the health care professional must be able to identify which babies are suitable for transitional care, if the service is available.

Transitional care means that separation of mother and baby is avoided, the mother has the opportunity to learn to care for the baby herself and is able to assume the role of mother. Transitional care has been shown to be very beneficial for moderately compromised neonates and their families (Duddridge, 2001). As there is no separation of mother and baby the ability of mothers to learn their baby's behavioural cues should be enhanced. The mother may also have an opportunity to learn the physical care of her baby, allowing her to gain confidence with the skills required when caring for a baby with special needs. When the mother returns home with her baby she should have greater confidence with her mother-ing skills than if she had been separated from her baby for long periods of time. The National Institute for Health and Clinical Excellence (NICE, 2006) recommend that hospitals should provide a good environment for women and their babies and should ensure round-the-clock rooming in, privacy, adequate rest and ready access to food and drink. This may be achieved by caring for mothers and babies within a dedicated transitional care ward. Offering transitional care to the woman and her baby is also in keeping with the *National Service Framework for Children, Young People and Maternity Services* to ensure that frontline services are built around the needs of children and their families (DH, 2004).

As a transition between hospital and home, neonatal outreach support may be offered to families. This enables babies who are well and main-taining their temperature, but who may require some gastric tube feeds, to go home with their parents at an earlier stage. Neonatal outreach support can support the family to ensure that feeds are given safely and to continue to monitor the babies' well-being and progress. The neonatal outreach team are often neonatal nurses with a post-registration qualification who work in close collaboration with the community midwife team to ensure the family receive optimum support. However, not all maternity/neonatal units offer this service.

Neonatal managed clinical networks

In 2003 the Government undertook a review of neonatal care services and, following this, introduced neonatal managed clinical networks (NMCN). These were developed to try to enable high-quality care to be given across wide geographical areas. Although they are mainly concerned with the care of sicker babies, it is important that the health care practitioner has a clear idea of how neonatal care is organised to ensure that the women and their babies receive the highest level of care.

The National Service Framework (NSF) define a managed neonatal care network as 'linked groups of health professionals and organisations from primary, secondary and tertiary care and social services and other services, working together in a co-ordinated manner, to ensure an equitable provision of high quality, clinically effective care' (DH, 2004). There are 24 NMCNs throughout England (NHS Neonatal Networks, 2008). The purpose of each NMCN is to try to ensure that mothers and their babies receive care within their own network and only occasionally from an adjacent NMCN. It was intended that this would enable babies to receive treatment close to their home (DH, 2003). The networks are also intended to ensure that an appropriate concentration of skills and expertise is available within each NMCN. The NSF (DH, 2004) says that the managed clinical networks should ensure that there are effective arrangements for the transfer of women and their babies needing specialist care.

It is important that you have an understanding of the different types of classification of babies, the type of care they may need and in which level of unit they may need to be cared for. This will help you to provide explanations for parents when they ask you questions in relation to the care their baby may need.

Key points
- Understanding classifications of babies is key to planning appropriate care to meet both their own and their parents' needs.
- Each baby should receive care depending upon its individual needs.
- The role of neonatal managed clinical networks may impact on the type of care available to the baby locally.

Exercises

1. You are the midwife working in the delivery suite. You have just delivered a baby who is 35 weeks' gestation and weighs 2.4 kg. What type of care might be suitable for this baby and why?

2. You are the midwife working in the delivery suite. You have just delivered a baby born at 39 weeks' gestation who weighs 3.5 kg. What type of care do you think this baby may need and why?
3. What are the benefits of transitional care and early discharge for mothers and their babies?

REFERENCES

BLISS (2004) *Community Health Professionals' Information Guide.* London: BLISS (the premature baby charity)

British Association of Perinatal Medicine (2001) *Standards for Hospitals Providing Neonatal Intensive and High Dependency Care* (2nd Ed.) and *Categories of Babies Requiring Neonatal Care.* London: BAPM

Bromley, P. (2000) 'Transitional care: let's think again'. *Journal of Neonatal Nursing* (6) 2: 60–64

Department of Health (2003) *Report of DH expert working group on Neonatal Intensive Care Services.* London: DH

Department of Health (2004) *National Service Framework for Children, Young People and Maternity Services.* London: DH

Duddridge, E. (2001) 'What are the advantages of transitional care for neonates?' *British Journal of Midwifery*, (9)2: 92–99

England, C. (2003) 'The healthy low birthweight baby', in Fraser, D. and Cooper, M. (eds) *Myles Textbook for Midwives* (14th Ed.). Edinburgh: Churchill Livingstone

Johnston, P., Flood, K. and Spinks, K. (2004) *The Newborn Child* (9th Ed.). Edinburgh: Churchill Livingstone

National Institute for Health and Clinical Excellence (NICE) (2006) *Routine postnatal care of women and their babies.* London: NICE

NHS Neonatal Networks (2008) at: **www.neonatal.org.uk/Healthcare+Professionals/About+the+Networks**

Nursing and Midwifery Council (2004) *Midwives rules and standards.* London: NMC

Papageorgiou, A. and Bardin, C. (1999) 'The extremely-low-birth-weight infant', in Avery, G., Fletcher, M. and Macdonald, M. (eds) *Neonatology-Pathophysiology and Management of the Newborn*. Philadelphia: Lippincott Williams and Wilkins

Stables, D. and Rankin, J. (2005) *Physiology in Childbearing with Anatomy and Related Biosciences*. Edinburgh: Elsevier

Viccars, A. (2003) 'Antenatal care' in Fraser, D. and Cooper, M. (eds) *Myles Textbook for Midwives* (14th Ed.). Edinburgh: Churchill Livingstone

Chapter 2

Maternal and Family Health and the Impact on the Fetus and Neonate

Mary Melley and Kenda Crozier

Chapter aims

This chapter will explore the significance of health promotion and public health issues in relation to maternal and family health.

Learning outcomes

At the end of this chapter you will be able to:

- discuss the importance of maternal and family health in relation to the growing fetus and neonate;
- examine the impact that maternal and family health may have on the neonate once born;
- discuss specific issues that may impact on the health of mother and fetus;
- demonstrate an understanding of the significance of family-centred health promotion activities.

Mapping to Standards of Proficiency

Standards of Proficiency for Pre-registration Midwifery Education (SPME)
Communicate with women and their families throughout the preconception, antenatal, intrapartum and postnatal periods, including:

- actively encouraging women to think about their own health and the health of their babies and families and how this can be improved;
- caring for and monitoring women during the puerperium, offering the necessary evidence-based advice and support regarding the baby and self-care, including enabling women to address their own and their babies' and their families' health and social well-being.

NHS Knowledge and Skills Framework (NHS KSF)
Core 5, Level 2

Standards of Proficiency for Pre-registration Nursing Education
- Consult with patients, clients and groups to identify their need and desire for health promotion advice.

> • Utilise a range of effective and appropriate communication and engagement skills.

INTRODUCTION

This chapter will explore the impact of the health of the mother on the development of the baby, both before and during pregnancy. We will discuss the impact of inequality on health outcomes for families and key areas in which health professionals can influence the health of families. The public health element of care is an integral part of midwifery practice and is clearly recognised in the activities of a midwife in the *Midwives Rules and Standards* (NMC, 2004). Nursery nurses and maternity or health care assistants also have an important role in giving health advice to women about the care of their babies.

What do we mean by public health?

Heller *et al.*, (2003) describe the use of population sciences, such as surveys, as a means of identifying the health needs of communities. This means that health is viewed by examining communities and societies as a whole to determine how specific interventions might be developed to improve the health of certain groups in society or the population as a whole. The focus of public health services often involves working at improving health among those communities where health inequalities are identified.

Inequalities in health are defined according to mortality (death) and morbidity (significant illness or disability) rates in relation to socio-economic status (Stringer, 2007). The fact of health inequality is quite a simple equation. The poorer you are in economic terms the more likely you are to suffer ill health (DH, 2003). Those living in the poorest areas often have less access to health care, and uptake of screening, immunisation and other public health services are reduced (Stringer, 2007). The Department of Health further identifies a lack of support networks, lack of confidence, lack of role models and very inflexible working patterns as issues that inhibit access to services in deprived areas (DH, 2005). *The National Service Framework for Children, Young People and Maternity Services* (DH, 2004a) aimed to address health inequalities and improve access to services for those most in need. The report emphasised the need for flexible services designed to fit around the journey through pregnancy and motherhood of the woman and her baby, with emphasis on the needs of vulnerable and disadvantaged women. It is important that the pregnancy and birth process follows a normal path and medical intervention should not be considered without a clinical indication (DH, 2004a). It is important that the promotion of family health should begin before conception.

PRECONCEPTION CARE

Preconception advice and care is about giving timely information to women that will enable them to make informed decisions about their health status and lifestyle habits before pregnancy. Preconception care is aimed at ensuring that both parents are in optimal health at the time of conception and during the period of organogenesis, thus increasing the chances of a healthy baby. Most major organs and organ systems are formed between the third and eighth week following conception. This critical period for normal development is known as organogenesis (Sadler, 2006).

Interventions such as immunisations and folic acid supplementation should begin at least three to six months before conception. For decades health professionals have discussed the need for preconception care and the benefits that it may bring. But it is still a struggle to reach the vulnerable groups who would benefit most from advice on pre-pregnancy health and preparation for pregnancy. Mental capacity and behavioural characteristics as well as physical well-being are affected during the development of the embryo and fetus. Factors such as maternal smoking, nutrition, drug and alcohol intake, stress and diabetes all impact on the future long-term health of the baby (Sadler, 2006). Those who are offered preconception advice at present tend to be women with pre-existing medical conditions such as diabetes, epilepsy and phenylketonuria (PKU).

Information box 1

What is PKU?
This condition is due to the deficiency of the enzyme Phenylalanine hydroxylase which coverts the amino acid phenylanine, found in most foods, into tyrosine. On establishing milk feeds the levels of phenylanine, together with the by product of its metabolism, phenylpyruvic acid, start to rise. Phenylpyruvic acid is toxic to the neonatal brain, causing irreversible neurological damage. Neonatal screening for this condition and the commencement of early phenylalanine-restricted diets has led to excellent outcomes. Women with PKU must begin the restricted diets before embarking on a pregnancy and maintain it throughout pregnancy to protect the fetus. See Chapter 4 for more information.

A new aspect of health that is emerging as an important area of concern in pregnancy is obesity. It is now a recognised high-risk factor in pregnancy (Confidential Enquiry into Maternal and Child Health, Lewis, 2007) so overweight women should seek advice on losing weight before embarking on a pregnancy. A recent study predicts that by 2010 as many as 22 per cent of women attending for antenatal booking could be obese. Obesity is 2.5 times greater in women from lower socio-economic backgrounds than in the general population (Heslehurst *et al.*, 2007).

Important preconception interventions for improving pregnancy outcomes

Folic acid supplementation: 400 µg per day for low-risk women; 5 mg per day for women considered to be at high risk.	Reduces occurrence of neural tube defects such as spina bifida by two thirds.
Rubella vaccination.	Congenital deafness may be prevented.
Smoking cessation.	May prevent low birth weight and preterm birth complications.
Stopping alcohol consumption.	Reduces risk of fetal alcohol syndrome.
Obesity control.	Reduces the risk of preterm birth and, in the mother, diabetes, hypertension and thromboembolic disorders such as deep vein thrombosis (DVT).
Careful dietary management of mothers with PKU.	Prevention of learning disabilities relating to PKU.
HIV screening.	Allows couples to make decisions about pregnancy and to commence treatment for prevention of mother-to-child transmission if necessary.
Diabetes management, control of blood sugar levels.	Reduces the risk of large babies and stillbirth.
Review of antiepileptic drugs.	This allows clinicians to change drug therapy to reduce the risk of harm to the fetus from the medication.

ANTENATAL CARE

The aim of antenatal care is to monitor the health of the mother and fetus to ensure that the pregnancy is progressing normally and to identify any deviations from the expected progress.

Providing antenatal care and advice to women is an integral part of the role of the midwife. But all health care practitioners who come into contact with women during pregnancy should consider the advice that can be given to improve health outcomes for mothers and babies.

> From a midwifery perspective antenatal care is not an independent entity. It is an integral part of the whole childbearing experience. It usually represents the beginning of the journey that midwives and women will make together which includes the time before, during and after the birth of the baby.
>
> (Grigg, 2006, p. 342)

The first meeting between a pregnant woman and the midwife forms the basis of an ongoing relationship. It is important that information is shared between them so that the midwife gains the important information needed to assess and plan care and so that the woman gains information to make decisions about her pregnancy screening tests and lifestyle choices. The midwife must take a detailed history and ascertain the date of the last menstrual period in order to work out the expected date of delivery and to arrange suitable screening tests at the most appropriate times. The medical history should include questions about operations and existing medical disease or conditions such as diabetes, hypertension, epilepsy, cardiac disorders and rheumatological conditions. Childhood illnesses should also be discussed and Rubella immunity status should be ascertained. Any history of mental illness is an important factor to note (this will be discussed in more detail later in this chapter). A family history is also important, especially in relation to genetic disorders so that specific screening and counselling may be offered. History of previous pregnancies is important, particularly where there were complications. The woman should be asked about drug use including prescribed medications and street drugs. The use of alcohol should be discussed in relation to fetal development and women should be encouraged to avoid alcohol, particularly in early pregnancy. Smoking needs to be addressed in a way that will enable the woman to feel supported in her attempts to cease tobacco use.

In relation to diet the woman should be advised about avoiding foods which may pose a bacteriological risk such as soft cheeses and foods that may contain listeria. The link between vitamin A in liver and congenital abnormalities should be highlighted so that women avoid this either as a dietary supplement or in liver products such as pâté.

Folic acid supplements should be offered to those women who have not commenced taking this supplement prior to pregnancy. These should be continued until the 12th week of pregnancy. The NICE (2007a) consultation document on antenatal care advises that vitamin D supplements should be considered for some women:

> Oral vitamin D supplement of 10 micrograms per day should be offered to healthy pregnant women at risk of vitamin D deficiency, for example women with dark skin, women who usually cover their skin, women who eat a vegan diet and women in age group 19–24 years.
>
> (NICE, 2007a, p. 6)

TEENAGE PREGNANCY AND HEALTH INEQUALITIES

It is generally recognised that teenage pregnancy and health inequalities are closely linked. The Government has set targets for the reduction of teenage pregnancies in England and local primary care trusts are working in many areas in a multiagency way to try to achieve this reduction (Department for Children, Schools and Families, 2007). From the work that has been done so far in this area the most successful strategies have included providing:

- services for young people with improved access to advice and support;
- education to provide knowledge, skills and confidence so that young people can be employed and thus avoid the poverty trap;
- sex education which sends strong messages about negative consequences of sex at an early age, i.e. unintended pregnancy, or HIV or other sexually transmitted infections;
- the facilitation of open discussion between parents and children;
- advice on contraception to young women with a prior conception.
                    (Department for Children, Schools and Families, 2007)

One in every ten babies born in England is to a teenage mother. These children are at high risk of growing up in poverty and experiencing poor health and social outcomes. The Independent Advisory Group (IAG) on Teenage Pregnancy was set up in 2000 to advise and implement a strategy on the teenage pregnancy (IAG on Teenage Pregnancy, 2002). The strategy has set a target of halving the number of teenage pregnancies by 2010. It also aims to increase the participation of teenagers in education, training and employment to address the issue of inequality.

Risks associated with teenage pregnancies

Babies of teenage mothers are more likely to be born preterm (that is before 37 completed weeks' gestation). There is a 25 per cent higher risk that the babies born to teenage mothers will have low birth weights. The lifestyle of teenagers is thought to be a contributing factor to many of the health problems of these babies. Teenage mothers are more likely to smoke and continue to smoke throughout pregnancy. They are also likely to suffer from poor nutrition (Lawler and Shaw, 2002). It is important that when dealing with pregnant teenagers you approach them with sensitivity and offer advice that is tailored to meet their needs. It is important not to make assumptions about their lifestyles but to ask sensitive questions and offer them the opportunity to discuss their own worries and concerns.

Teenagers tend to book later for antenatal care, according to the Department for Children, Schools and Families (2007). The average for a teenager is 16 weeks. The latest CEMACH (Confidential Enquiry into Maternal and Child Health, Lewis, 2007) report has identified that 17 per cent of those mothers who died in pregnancy and during the first year after giving birth had booked late or missed more than four routine antenatal visits. This can be attributed to a number of factors, including difficulty of access to antenatal clinics, fear of judgement by midwives and older mothers, and a lack of understanding about pregnancy and the importance of antenatal care. Teenage mothers are less likely to breastfeed than older mothers. Teenage risk-taking behaviour also includes the misuse of substances and alcohol. Teenagers who become pregnant have a higher risk of hypertension, depression and isolation (Lawlor and Shaw, 2002). These factors all have a long-term impact on their future health and well-being and that of their babies.

The figures quoted express the serious issue to be addressed in meeting the needs of teenagers and addressing these early. Therefore, preconception education is of great importance in this age group. Sex education programmes in schools need to include discussion of preparation for pregnancy and parenthood in terms of general health as well as readiness in relation to maturity and relationship choices. It is important therefore that school nurses and others who work with young people in family planning centres and other health settings are able to discuss maternal health with young people.

DIABETES

The St Vincent declaration of 1989, which was a joint statement by all European governments, stated that pregnancy outcomes for women with diabetes should differ little from those without diabetes. NICE guidelines (2008a) set standards for the care of diabetic women of childbearing age.

Information box 2

Diabetes

Diabetes is a disorder of carbohydrate metabolism that requires immediate changes in lifestyle. In its chronic forms, diabetes is associated with long-term vascular complications, including retinopathy, nephropathy, neuropathy and vascular disease. (NICE, 2008a). The following are the classifications of diabetes described by the World Health Organization in 1999.

- **Type 1** (caused by beta-cell destruction, usually leading to absolute insulin deficiency). Can be either autoimmune or idiopathic. Characterised by poor control of blood sugar and high levels of blood sugar even after fasting (a level of 7 mmol/l or more after fasting, and greater than 11.1 mmol/l at two hours following a 75 g dose of glucose, is used for diagnosis). Patients with type 1 diabetes require regular insulin injections for survival.
- **Type 2** is the most common form of diabetes and is characterised by disorders of insulin action and insulin secretion, either of which may be the predominant feature. Both are usually present at the time that this form of diabetes is clinically manifest. Not all patients with type 2 diabetes will require insulin therapy. This type of diabetes is commonly associated with obesity.

Gestational diabetes

To determine if gestational diabetes is present in pregnant women, a standard Glucose Tolerance Test should be performed after overnight fasting (8–14 hours) by giving 75 g anhydrous glucose in 250–300 ml water. Plasma glucose is measured fasting and after two hours in pregnant women who meet WHO criteria for diabetes mellitus or are classified as having Gestational Diabetes Mellitus (GDM).

Preconception care for women with diabetes is vitally important because those women with poor glycaemic (blood sugar) control before pregnancy will also have poor glycaemic control during pregnancy. Therefore it is important that the condition is well controlled and the woman feels confident in self-management before pregnancy begins (Lewis, 2007). Diabetic women should be encouraged to plan their pregnancies carefully. During pregnancy these women should be cared for by a multidisciplinary team including midwives, obstetricians and diabetes specialists. Diabetes specialist midwives often act as the co-ordinator of care for pregnant diabetics, linking with other members of the multidisciplinary team.

Type 1 and type 2 diabetes together account for one in 250 pregnancies (Macfarlane and Tuffnell, 2006) and it is thought that the rise in diabetes in the UK population may be associated with the epidemic of obesity. In young women the rise in obesity and the subsequent diabetes impacts upon their own health and the health of their babies (Saad *et al.*, 2005). Women who embark on pregnancy with inadequate glycaemia control risk pregnancy complications including miscarriage and perinatal death, babies with neural tube defects, such as spina bifida, and also an increased risk of babies with heart defects (Pearson *et al.*, 2007). To prevent neural tube defects in babies of diabetic mothers, folic acid 5 mg per day should be commenced in the preconception period (Lumley *et al.*, 2006).

Women with diabetes require careful monitoring throughout pregnancy but particularly during delivery. Their babies need to be monitored for the risk of developing hypoglycaemia following birth (see Chapter 8). Each hospital trust will have a policy for the care of babies of diabetic mothers.

The midwife can use the postnatal period as an opportunity to discuss the importance of preconception care for future pregnancies in those women who have experienced diabetes in pregnancy.

SMOKING IN PREGNANCY

In the UK, Department of Health statistics show that 120 000 preventable illnesses a year are linked to smoking, including one third of all perinatal deaths (DH, 2004b). Smoking impacts on the fetus in a number of ways. Nicotine is a vasoconstrictor so may restrict placental blood flow, which in turn may lead to growth restriction in the fetus. Babies born to smokers are more likely to be of low birth weight as a result. Carbon monoxide binds to haemoglobin, which is the oxygen-carrying component of blood. Therefore, less oxygen may be supplied to the fetus. Babies born to smokers weigh on average 200–250 g less than babies of non-smokers. There is a relationship between the number of cigarettes smoked and the birth weight so the more the mother smokes the lighter the baby. Low birth weight in these babies may be as a result of growth restriction but also preterm birth is more common in babies of smokers (British Medical Association (BMA), 2004).

Information box 3

The effects of smoking on pregnancy
- There is an increased risk of ectopic pregnancy and miscarriage.
- Smokers are three times more likely to have a low birth weight baby.
- Smokers are more likely to give birth prematurely.

- Smokers are more likely to suffer stillbirth.
- Babies born to smokers are more likely to die within the first four weeks of life.
- Placental complications such as placental abruption and placenta praevia are more common in the smoker.
- Increased risk of fetal malformations such as cleft lip and palate may be associated with smoking.

(BMA, 2004)

Women who stop smoking before becoming pregnant are less likely to resume than those who stop during pregnancy. Seventy per cent of women who stopped smoking when they found out they were pregnant had resumed smoking by six months after the birth (Lumley *et al.*, 2002).

Information box 4

The effects of smoking on infant and child health (BMA, 2004)
- Babies may suffer nicotine withdrawal symptoms.
- There is an increased risk of cot death.
- Children of smokers have poorer lung function than children of non-smokers.
- Children who are subjected to passive smoking may develop asthma and the attacks may be more severe.
- Babies born to smokers are smaller and lighter as children.
- Compared to children of non-smokers, children of smokers have poorer scores at school, shorter attention span and behavioural problems.
- In adult life these children may be at greater risk of developing cardiovascular disease and impaired lung function.

Smoking cessation in pregnancy

All midwives should receive training in how to help pregnant women to stop smoking. But all health professionals should be able to discuss the risks of smoking in pregnancy and be able to listen to women's worries and concerns regarding smoking. Midwives must address the issue of smoking at the first antenatal appointment or in a preconception clinic. Women need to be given clear, accurate information about the risks of smoking during pregnancy to the woman and her fetus. It is important that women are referred for specialist smoking cessation counselling because smoking cessation programmes during pregnancy appear to reduce smoking, according to Lumley *et al.*, (2002). Stopping smoking at any time in pregnancy is of benefit to the fetus so you should always encourage all attempts on the part of the woman to stop. Health professionals should show an empathetic approach rather than being judgemental, and demonstrate some understanding of the difficulties of giving up smoking. You also should consider that smoking is a coping mechanism for other issues in the lives of some women (Heggie, 2006). Allow women to talk about their reasons for smoking and try to help them consider ways to stop smoking. Women who are pregnant can use the nicotine substitute patches to help them. However, they should seek advice on their use as, according to NHS guidance, it is inadvisable to wear the patches at night when pregnant.

ALCOHOL AND PREGNANCY

Alcohol consumption during pregnancy is a major public health concern because of potential adverse long-term physical, neurodevelopment and behavioural consequences for children (Mukherjee *et al.*, 2005). Recent advice in a BMA report recommends that abstinence is the only safe policy for women who are pregnant or planning a pregnancy (BMA, 2007). This view is shared by the Royal College of Obstetricians and Gynaecologists (RCOG, 2006) and the World Health Organization (WHO, 2006). Controversially, the National Institute for Health and Clinical Excellence advised that 'pregnant women should limit their alcohol intake to less than one standard drink (1.5 UK units of alcohol) per day and if possible avoid alcohol in the first three months of pregnancy' (NICE, 2008b). These mixed messages can cause confusion among women about the safety of alcohol in pregnancy and increase anxiety levels.

For centuries, observations all over the world have shown that maternal drinking during pregnancy can have serious adverse effects on the newborn. However, it was not until 1967, in France, that Lemoine and his team first described in scientific terms a group of children affected by maternal alcohol abuse, which included impaired intrauterine and postpartum growth, unusual facial features, congenital malformations, such as cardiac defects, and cleft palate combined with mental 'subnormality' (Lemoine *et al.*, 1968).

Fetal alcohol syndrome

The term Fetal Alcohol Spectrum Disorder (FASD) is used to describe a wide spectrum of adverse effects on the fetus associated with maternal drinking during pregnancy, the most dramatic of which is Fetal Alcohol

Syndrome (FAS). Because the fetus does not have a blood filtration system, it is unprotected from alcohol in the bloodstream (Nathanson *et al.*, 2007). Effects seen in a child, and the diagnosis reached, depend on the duration of exposure to substantial maternal alcohol consumption during pregnancy, the range and timing of peak blood alcohol levels, the nutritional state of the mother, use of other drugs (including tobacco), general health of the mother, stress, maternal age and low socioeconomic status (Mukherjee *et al.*, 2006; O'Leary, 2005). Characteristics which may lead to a diagnosis of fetal alcohol syndrome include the following:

- abnormalities of growth, including low birth weight and small head circumference;
- central nervous system involvement;
- small, widely spaced eyes, flat midface, short, upturned nose, thin upper lip;
- babies are irritable and have trouble with eating and sleeping;
- babies are sensitive to sensory stimulation, which can include distress when being held or cuddled, and have a strong startle reflex. They may have either high or low muscle tone.

It is claimed that the neurological and behavioural effects are frequently misdiagnosed as Attention Deficit Hyperactivity Disorder (ADHD) and not always connected to a diagnosis of FAS (Fryer *et al.*, 2007). Most children will have some developmental delays and some degree of learning difficulty. The features of FAS include:

- attention and memory deficits;
- hyperactivity;
- difficulty learning from behaviours;
- reduced problem-solving skills;
- difficulty with social functioning.

(Fryer *et al.*, 2007)

Drinking, especially binge-drinking, is increasing among women of child-bearing age in the UK and this may eventually lead to the birth of an even higher number of children with FAS – a major concern for the future. To improve the health, performance and social outcomes of such children and their mothers, the only safe message for women who are pregnant or planning a pregnancy must be complete abstinence from alcohol. Countries such as the USA, Canada, France, New Zealand and Australia have adopted this policy (Nathanson *et al.*, 2007).

Alcohol-induced fetal damage is totally preventable and, by informing both prospective parents of the potential dangers of alcohol consumption before conception, and particularly all women during pregnancy, we can hope to control the problem. The goal of public health education in this area should be not only to inform but also to create a climate of opinion in which abstinence during pregnancy is socially accepted behaviour.

SUBSTANCE MISUSE

Eleven per cent of those women who died in pregnancy and during the first year after giving birth in the period 2003–2005 had a history of substance misuse (Lewis, 2007). Drug misuse in pregnancy can have an effect on the development of the fetus and also long-term consequences for children. Some effects may be physical but the most important ones will be on the brain of the child. These effects may not be visible and, in some cases, the impact on the child's development and behaviour may not manifest itself for some years (Merredew, 2007). Although damage to the fetus can occur at any stage of the pregnancy, the first three months constitute the most vulnerable period for congenital malformations, while brain growth is most rapid in late pregnancy.

Cannabis is one of the most commonly used drugs in pregnant women, but little is known about its effects during pregnancy. One long-term study found that the speech or memory performance among four-year-olds whose mothers had consumed cannabis during pregnancy was affected significantly (Merredew, 2007).

The early reports on prenatal cocaine effects in the 1980s created a public frenzy and a myth about the 'dangerous' and 'unfit to parent' women and their damaged crack babies (Mayes *et al.*, 1992). Recent studies (Bauer *et al.*, 2005) have failed to support any association between prenatal cocaine exposure and increased prevalence of newborn serious congenital abnormalities.

Neonates whose mothers have used heroin may suffer withdrawal symptoms which may last up to several months and include tremors, high muscle tone, irritability, diarrhoea, vomiting and abnormal feeding and sleep patterns.

It is very hard to establish a diagnosis in babies and young children as being affected by parental drug abuse, and difficult also to diagnose the outcomes. This is partly due to the lack of conclusive research to date and also to the fact that it is nearly impossible to determine accurately the type, amount and timing in pregnancy for each substance used, especially as users often combine different drugs, sometimes with alcohol and often with tobacco. The chaotic lifestyles of those women who abuse a range of substances make them one of the vulnerable groups of women who need special care and attention in pregnancy. This involves a range of approaches from a multidisciplinary perspective, including the provision of help with housing, withdrawal programmes and benefits. Social services involvement may be needed if other children have already been deemed at risk.

DOMESTIC ABUSE

Domestic violence is defined as:

> Any violence between current or former partners in an intimate relationship wherever and when ever the violence occurs. The violence may include physical, sexual, emotional or financial abuse.
>
> (Walby and Allen, 2004, p. 4)

Domestic violence or domestic abuse has a devastating and lasting impact on families. However, the subject remains taboo and, because of the nature of the abuse, occurring behind closed doors, it is sometimes difficult to address the issue (Buck and Collins, 2007). Although women can be violent towards men in relationships, and domestic abuse also occurs within homosexual and lesbian relationships, statistically the most frequently reported occurrence is where women are the victims of male abuse (Aston, 2006). Fourteen per cent of the women whose deaths were reported during the period 2003–2005 had stated that they were subject to domestic abuse (Lewis, 2007). Ten per cent lived in families who were known to child protection services. It is important that the midwife is able to ask the woman about abuse in the home or partner abuse or domestic violence. All midwives should receive training in addressing the issue and be able to give women advice and information about where help can be obtained. The questions about domestic abuse should never be asked in the presence of the partner. Women may confide in other health care professionals who they think will be sympathetic. It is important that if a woman confides in you, you must discuss with her who you can share this information with. The CEMACH report also found that large numbers of women in abusive relationships had difficulty in maintaining contact with maternity services. Often the domineering partner disrupted the relationship between the woman and the health care providers.

Pregnancy can be a high-risk time when domestic abuse either begins or intensifies, with 30 per cent of domestic abuse starting in pregnancy (Mezey et al., 2002). Dealing with domestic violence requires a multi-agency approach, including the health professional, social services, the police and voluntary agencies. Midwives and other professionals caring for pregnant women need to be able to make contact with the relevant agencies where concern is aroused. Midwives should offer advice on how women can keep themselves safe and provide them with contacts for local services and agencies. The Metropolitan Police Service Domestic Violence Risk Assessment Model SPECCs (2003) is one model that may be helpful in planning multi agency approaches.

Women in abusive relationships may use tobacco, alcohol and other substances as a means of coping with the difficult situation. So, once again, it is important that you approach women disclosing the use of these substances with sensitivity.

MENTAL HEALTH IN PREGNANCY

Detecting problems

Ensuring good physical, social and emotional outcomes from pregnancy and childbirth are all-important in providing a healthy start to family life. The National Health Service Plan (DH, 2000) has identified mental health services for women as a priority area. Government guidelines stress the need for mental health problems to be detected and treated in pregnancy (NICE, 2007b) and the midwife can act as a key professional in the risk assessment and identification of needs (Hammond and Crozier, 2007). The maternity support worker who has contact with pregnant women or the nursery nurse who may be in contact with a family in the early postnatal period may also be in a position to identify those women at need. A simple process is recommended for the detection of problems. Women should be asked, at the first meeting with a midwife in the antenatal period, about family history of mental health problems, whether they have any history of mental health problems and whether they have received medication for these. They should be asked if they have been under the care of the mental health services, including care by community psychiatric nurses and psychiatrists. If they have received any care or treatment then the health records from the General Practitioner (GP) should be accessed for further information.

> **Information box 5**
>
> **Mental health**
> The questions that should be asked early in pregnancy (usually at the first appointment with the midwife) and at least twice in the postnatal period are:
>
> - during the past month have you often been bothered by feeling down, depressed or hopeless?

- during the past month have you often felt bothered by having little interest or pleasure in doing things?

If the answer to either question is yes, then:

- is this something you feel you need or want help with?

Other social or psychological indicators, according to Borthwick *et al.* (2004), which may be considered when assessing risk in pregnant women are:

- previous history of depression;
- current symptoms of depression;
- lack of social support;
- recent history of stressful life event (such as the death of a loved one);
- lack of confiding relationship;
- domestic abuse.

(Mezey *et al.*, 2005)

Care planning

There should be a clear referral route so that midwives and others, including health visitors and GPs, are able to communicate with mental health professionals who can arrange assessment for the woman. Good interprofessional communication is essential and yet it is clear that mental health services for women in pregnancy and in the postnatal period are not readily available in many localities in the UK (NICE, 2007b). The leading causes of maternal death (death during pregnancy or in the first year after birth) are those related to psychiatric disorders, including suicide (Lewis, 2007). Women who are taking medication for severe depression or any other mental health problem should continue to take this and be referred to the person who prescribed the medication for further advice. There needs to be careful planning for labour and also for the postnatal period as a mental health crisis may occur in the early postnatal period (NICE, 2007b). Therefore, women who are at risk should be visited on a daily basis by the community midwife to provide support for the woman and her family. Information should be given to the family so that they may be aware of signs of problems arising and seek appropriate help as early as possible. Planning for birth and postnatal care therefore needs to include the woman, her family, the midwife and other professionals such as the GP, psychiatric nurse or psychiatrist. Postnatal depression can occur in 10–20 per cent of women and, of these, 23 per cent of women revealed that their symptoms had begun in the antenatal period (NICE, 2007b).

Impact on the baby

Women with depression in pregnancy are more likely to smoke and misuse alcohol or substances (Zuckerman *et al.*, 1989). These are known to have negative effects on the growth and development of the fetus. Children of women who have had antenatal depression and postnatal depression have been found in research to have difficulties with behaviour in later life (O'Connor *et al.*, 2002). Women who have suffered depression in pregnancy and the postnatal period may have problems in bonding with their baby and this has been shown to impact on the educational attainment of children.

Many of the potential public health issues in pregnancy are interlinked and the influence of social inequality is an important consideration. Midwives and others working in maternity services should be aware of the social make-up of the communities in which they work. Problems faced by these communities can then be addressed on an individual level with women before, during and after pregnancy. Local knowledge and sensitive approaches to care planning and advice are important skills that can be developed over time. The importance of public health issues in pregnancy cannot be overestimated when you consider that these issues affect not only the present but future generations.

Key points
- Poverty and health inequalities are linked.
- Teenage pregnancy is an important area to be addressed in terms of social and health inequalities.
- Women with pre-existing medical conditions should be enabled to plan their pregnancies.
- Women who smoke should be given clear advice on the risks to their own and their baby's health and referred to specialist services to help them to stop smoking.
- Pregnancy is a risk factor for domestic abuse, and health care professionals should be able to ask women about this and give advice on where help can be offered.

Exercises

1. At the booking clinic 14-year-old Michaela has arrived unannounced and wants to see a midwife. She says that she is pregnant and her last period was three months ago. What are the issues of concern about this girl and what advice might be given to her by the midwife?

2. You are dealing with a client who discloses that she is using cannabis and occasionally 'other stuff'. Who else might be involved in the care of this client and what health concerns are there?
3. The woman who has come to see the midwife is 32 weeks pregnant and you are helping in the antenatal clinic. She says that she is feeling very low and has felt very unhappy for the last few weeks. Consider the impact of depression in pregnancy and how this might be addressed.

REFERENCES

Aston, G. (2006) 'Domestic violence and health promotion: midwives can make a difference', in Bowden, J. and Manning, V. (eds) *Health Promotion in Midwifery: principles and Practice* (2nd Ed.). London: Hodder Arnold

Bauer, C.R., Langer, J.C. and Shankaran, S. (2005) 'Acute neonatal effects of cocaine exposure during pregnancy'. *Archives of Pediatrics and Adolescent Medicine* 159: 824–834

Borthwick, R., Macleod, A. and Stanley, N. (2004) *Antenatal Depression: Developing an Effective and Coordinated Service Response*. The University of Hull, West Hull NHS Primary Care Trust

British Medical Association (2004) *Smoking and Reproductive life: the impact of smoking on sexual, reproductive and child health*. **www.bma.org. uk**

British Medical Association. (2007) *Fetal alcohol spectrum disorders*. London: BMA

Buck, L. and Collins, S. (2007) 'Why don't midwives ask about domestic abuse?' *British Journal of Midwifery*, 15 (2): 753–757

Department for Children, Schools and Families (2007) *Teenage Parents: next steps*. London: HMSO

Department of Health (2000) *The NHS Plan*. London: HMSO

Department of Health (2003) *Tackling health inequalities: a programme for action*. London: HMSO

Department of Health (2004a) *The National Service Framework for Children, Young People and Maternity Services*. London: DH

Department of Health (2004b) 'Summary of intelligence on tobacco' www.dh.gov.uk/en/publicationsandstatistics/publications/publications policyandguidance/DH_4094612

Department of Health (2005) *Tackling Health inequalities*. Status Report. London: DH

Fryer, S.L., McGee, C.C., Matt, G.E., Riley, E.P. and Mattson, S. N. (2007) 'Evaluation of psycopathological conditions in children with heavy prenatal alcohol exposure'. *Pediatrics*, 119 (3): 733–741

Grigg, C. (2006) 'Working with women in pregnancy', in Pairman, S., Pincombe, J., Thorogood, C. and Tracy, S. *Midwifery Preparation for Practice*. Edinburgh: Churchill Livingstone

Hammond, S. and Crozier, K. (2007) 'Depression: assessing the causes'. *Midwives: Journal of the Royal College of Midwives*, 10 (8): 365–367

Heggie, M.M. (2006) 'Smoking, pregnancy and the midwife' in Bowden, J. and Manning, V. (eds) *Health Promotion in Midwifery: Principles and Practice* (2nd Ed.). London: Hodder Arnold

Heller, R. F., Heller, T.D. and Pattison, S. (2003) 'Putting the public back into public health: part 2, How can public health be accountable to the public?' *Public Health*, 117 (1): 66–71

Heslehurst, N., Ells, L. J., Simpson, H., Batterham, A., Wilkinson, J. and Summerbell, C. D. (2007) 'Trends in maternal obesity incidence rates, demographic predictors and health inequalities in 36 821 women over a 15-year period'. *BJOG*, 114 (2): 187–94

Independent Advisory Group on Teenage Pregnancy. *First Annual Report of the Independent Advisory Group on Teenage Pregnancy*. London: HMSO

Lawlor, D. and Shaw, M. (2002) 'Too much too young: teenage pregnancy is not a public health problem'. *International Journal of Epidemiology*, 31: 552–554

Lemoine, P., Harousseau, H., Borteyru, J.-P. and Menuet, J.-C. (1968) cited in Tuula E. Tourmaa, *The Adverse Effects Of Alcohol on Reproduction* (booklet) www.foresight-preconception.org.uk/booklet_alcohol.htm (accessed 3 February 2008)

Lewis, G. (Ed.) (2007) The Confidential Enquiry into Maternal and Child Health (CEMACH) *Saving Mothers' Lives: reviewing maternal deaths to make motherhood safer – 2003–2005. The Seventh Report on Confidential Enquiries into Maternal Deaths in the United Kingdom.* London: CEMACH

Lumley, J., Watson, L., Watson, M. and Bower, C. (2006) 'Periconceptional supplementation with folate and/or multivitamins for preventing neural tube defects'. *Cochrane Pregnancy and Childbirth Group* (Cochrane Database of systematic reviews). *The Cochrane Library* 3.

Lumley, J., Oliver, S. and Waters, E. (2002) 'Interventions for promoting smoking cessation during pregnancy' *(Cochrane Review). The Cochrane Library* 1.

Macfarlane, A. and Tuffnell, D. (2006) 'Diabetes in Pregnancy'. *British Medical Journal,* 333 (7560): 157–158

Mayes, L.C., Granger, R.H., Bornstein, M.H. and Zuckerman, B. (1992) 'The problem of prenatal cocaine exposure. A rush to judgement'. *Journal of the Americal Medical Association,* 267: 406–408.

Merredew, F.(2007) Prenatal exposure to drugs and alcohol **www.bemy parent.org.uk/features/prenatal-exposure-to-drugs-and-alcohol,75.AR. html** (accessed 3 February 2008).

Metropolitan Police Service. *Metropolitan Police Service Domestic Violence Risk Assessment Model.* SPECCS. London: MPS 2003

Mezey, G., Bacchus, L., Bewley, S. and Haworth, A. (2002) *An exploration of the Prevalence, Nature and Effects of Domestic Violence in Pregnancy.* Violence Research Programme: Economic and Social Research Council

Mezey, G., Bacchus, L. and Bewley, S. (2005) 'Domestic violence, lifetime trauma and psychological health of childbearing women'. *BJOG,* 112: 197–204

Mukherjee, R.A., Hollins, S., Abou-Saleh, M.T. and Turk, J. (2005). 'Low level alcohol consumption and the fetus'. *British Medical Journal,* 330: 375–376

Mukherjee, R.A., Hollins, S. and Turk, J. (2006) 'Fetal alcohol spectrum disorder: an overview'. *Journal of the Royal Society of Medicine,* 99: 298–302

Nathanson, V., Jayesinghe, N. and Roycroft, R. (2007) 'Is it all right for women to drink small amounts of alcohol in pregnancy?' *British Medical Journal*, 335: 857

NICE (2007a) *Antenatal care guidelines*. Draft consultation document. **www.nice.org.uk/nicemedia/pdf/ANCpartialupdate2008Version.pdf**

NICE (2007b) *Antenatal and postnatal mental health guidelines*. **www. nice.org**

NICE (2008) NICE clinical guideline 63, *Diabetes in pregnancy: management of diabetes and its complications from pre-conception to the postnatal period*. National Collaborating Centre for Women's and Children's Health.

NICE (2008b) *Antenatal Care: routine care for the healthy pregnant woman* (2nd Ed.) **www.nice.org.uk/guidance**

Nursing and Midwifery Council (2004) *Midwives rules and standards*. London: NMC

O'Connor, T.G., Heron, J., Golding, J., Beveridge, M. and Glover, V. (2002) 'Maternal antenatal anxiety and children's behavioural problems at four years'. *British Journal of Psychiatry*, 180: 502–508

O'Leary, C.M. (2005) 'Fetal alcohol syndrome: diagnosis, epidemiology, and development outcomes'. *Journal of Paediatric and Child Health*, 40: 2–7.

Pearson, D.W., Kernaghan, D., Lee, R. and Penney, G.C. (2007) 'The relationship between pre-pregnancy care and early pregnancy loss, major congenital anomaly or perinatal death in Type 1 diabetes mellitus'. *BJOG*, 114 (1): 104–107

Royal College of Obstetricians and Gynaecologists (2006) *Alcohol and Pregnancy –information for you*. **www.rcog.org.uk/resources/public/pdf/ alcohol_pregnancy_1206.pdf** (accessed 3 February 2008)

Saad, R., Gunger, N. and Arslanian, S. (2005) 'Progression from normal glucose tolerance to type 2 diabetes in a young girl: longitudinal changes in insulin sensitivity and secretion assessed by the clamp technique and surrogate estimates'. *Pediatric Diabetes*, 6 (2): 95–99

Sadler, T.W. (2006) *Langmans' Medical Embryology* (10th Ed.). Baltimore: Lippincott, Williams and Wilkins

Stringer, E. (2007) 'Health and Inequality', in Edwards, G. and Byrom, S. *Essential Midwifery Practice: Public Health.* Oxford: Blackwell Publishing

Walby, S. and Allen, J. (2004) *Domestic violence, sexual assault and stalking: findings from the British Crime Survey.* Home Office Research Study 276. London: Home Office Research, Development and Statistics Directorate

World Health Organization (1999) *Definition, Diagnosis and Classification of Diabetes Mellitus and its Complications.* Geneva: WHO

World Health Organization (2006) *Framework for alcohol policy in the WHO European Region.* Denmark: WHO Regional Office for Europe.

Zuckerman, Amar. H., Bauchner, H. and Cabral, H. (1989) 'Depressive symptoms during pregnancy: relationships to poor health behaviors'. *American Journal of Obstetrics and Gynecology* 160; 110–111

Useful websites

www.everychildmatters.gov.uk

www.bemyparent.org.uk/features/prenatal-exposure-to-drugs-andalco hol,75,AR.html (accessed 13 February 2008)

Chapter 3

Transition to Extrauterine Life
Amanda Williamson

Chapter aims

To introduce the student to the physiological changes that occur to a fetus at birth and the role of the nurse or midwife in assisting the neonate to make this effective transition.

Learning outcomes

By the end of this chapter you will be able to:

- demonstrate a working knowledge of the physiological transition from fetus to neonate;
- identify the immediate needs of the neonate and discuss ways in which the midwife or nurse can ensure that these needs are met;
- describe neonatal resuscitation, thermoregulation and vitamin K administration.

Mapping to standards of proficiency

Standards of Proficiency for Pre-registration Midwifery Education
Undertake appropriate emergency procedures to meet the health needs of women and babies. Emergency procedures will include:

- resuscitation of . . . baby.

Examine and care for babies immediately following birth. This will include:

- confirming their vital signs and taking the appropriate action.

Standards of Proficiency for Pre-registration Nursing Education
- Analyse and revise expected outcomes, nursing interventions and priorities in accordance with changes in the individual's condition, needs or circumstances.
- Recognise the need for adaptation and adapt nursing practice to meet varying and unpredictable circumstances.

INTRODUCTION

While it was growing inside its mother the baby only had to make minimal effort in order to meet its needs. The baby's needs for oxygenation, thermoregulation, nutrition and excretion were all met by its mother via the placenta. We will consider each of these needs and the effective transition the baby must make in this chapter.

Once the baby is born it needs to make a dramatic transition to ensure its survival. Most babies make a smooth transition to extrauterine life but not all do. As a health care practitioner caring for babies, you need to understand the processes of this transition so that you are able to give the baby appropriate care. You will be able to understand the reasons behind the care the baby needs and be able to explain that care to parents.

TRANSITION

Cardiovascular and respiratory

Obviously the most vital and important transition the baby makes is that related to airway and breathing. Without adequate oxygenation of vital organs the baby will not survive.

Fetal circulation

In order to understand the transition the baby makes, it is important that you understand the principles of fetal circulation. Fetal circulation is different from that of adult (newborn) circulation and there are four major differences that you should be aware of to ensure you understand the adaptation the baby must make at birth. You may need to read this section a few times before you understand it.

Summary of fetal circulation (See Figure 3.1)

- The umbilical vein (1) carries oxygenated blood from the placenta to the liver.
- The ductus venosus (2) branches from the umbilical vein and transmits a greater amount of oxygenated blood into the inferior vena cava (3).
- The hepatic vein leaves the liver and also returns blood to the inferior vena cava (3).
- The inferior vena cava (3) then carries this blood to the right atrium of the heart (4).
- The foramen ovale (5) allows most of the oxygenated blood to pass from the right atrium to the left atrium (6).

- This blood then passes through the mitral valve (7) to the left ventricle (8) leaving the heart through the ascending aorta (9) to supply the head and upper extremities.
- This means that the liver, heart and brain receive the best supply of oxygenated blood.
- The superior vena cava (10) returns blood from the head and upper extremities to the right atrium (4). This then passes through the tricuspid valve (11) into the right ventricle (12).
- The pulmonary artery (13) shunts some of this mixed blood to the non-functioning lungs.
- The ductus arteriosus (14) shunts most of the blood from the right ventricle (12) directly into the descending aorta (15) to supply the abdomen, pelvis and lower extremities.
- The hypogastric arteries (16) carry blood back to the placenta.

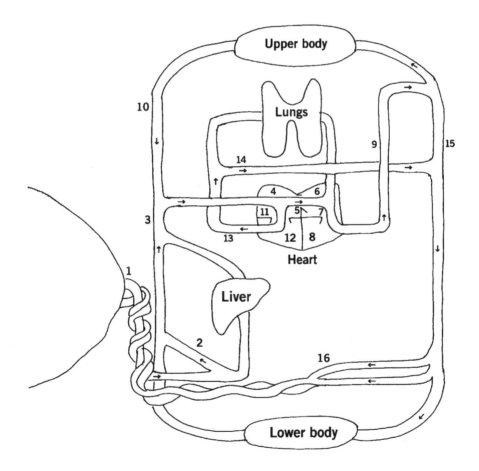

Figure 3.1 Diagram of fetal circulation

Fetal respiration (breathing)

As said previously the fetus in the uterus has obtained oxygen and excreted its carbon dioxide via the placenta. The fetus may have breathing movements noted on ultrasound from the first 12 weeks of pregnancy (Coad and Dunstall, 2005). Although the lungs are not used, the movements are thought to be important as they promote growth and allow the fetus to 'practise' breathing movements (Tucker Blackburn, 2003). The fetal lungs contain fluid, some of which will be expelled during chest compression throughout delivery (Johnston et al., 2004). When a woman is in labour, it is thought that the production of adrenaline by the fetus and thyrotophin-releasing hormone by the mother encourages the cells responsible for releasing fluid to stop, and for fluid to be absorbed from the alveolar spaces in the lungs in preparation for extrauterine life (Resuscitation Council UK, 2006).

The fetus receives intermittent reduction of oxygen during contractions, which leads to some fetal hypoxia (low oxygen levels) (Resuscitation Council UK, 2006). It is vital that, once the cord is cut at delivery, respiration is established as the lungs and not the placenta become the site of gaseous exchange (Fraser Askin, 2002). The respiratory system must be intact for this to occur successfully.

Transition of the cardiovascular and respiratory system at birth

Respiration

If you have seen any babies born you may have noticed that they generally make a loud and lusty cry. Most babies born at term will breathe or cry within 90 seconds of birth (Resuscitation Council UK, 2006). This lusty cry is very important as it generates a very high negative intrathoracic pressure that is usually required to initially inflate the lungs at birth (like taking a large deep breath). This may be as high as 60 cm of water but is usually thought to be between 20 and 30 cms of water (Johnston et al., 2004). After this initial breath a lower pressure (of about 5 cm water) is then required as the presence of a substance called surfactant in the lungs reduces surface tension in the alveoli (Johnston et al., 2004). The presence of surfactant in the lungs prevents the collapse of alveoli once they have been inflated. The baby's breathing rate will normally be between 40 to 60 breaths per minute (Fraser, 2003). If the baby has a breathing rate that is higher than 60 breaths per minute you may need to call for a paediatrician to review the baby. You would expect the baby's breathing pattern to be irregular and the baby may have periodic breathing periods (vigorous breaths followed by up to a 20-second pause) (Fraser Askin, 2002). The baby's breathing should be diaphragmatic chest and abdominal, they are obligatory nose breathers (Farrell and Sittlington, 2003).

Circulation

When the cord is cut, major changes occur to allow blood to be diverted to the lungs rather than to the placenta for oxygenation. It may be worth reading this in conjunction with Figure 3.1 above so that you are able to track the changes.

- With the first breath the lungs expand and more blood flows through the pulmonary arteries to the lungs (rather than into the ductus arteriosus (14) which bypassed the lungs).
- With increasing oxygenation the pulmonary vascular resistance reduces and this in turn initiates the closure of the ductus arteriosus.
- Increased blood volume from the lungs returns to the heart, thereby increasing the pressure in the left atrium (6) (this assists in closing the flap-like valve – the foramen ovale (5) – between the two atria).The flow of blood from the right to the left atrim through the foramen ovale ceases.
- The vessels that had carried deoxygenated blood to the placenta, the hypogastric arteries (16) and oxygenated blood from the placenta to the fetus (umbilical vein and ductus venosus (1and 2)) close and eventually become ligaments.
- These changes occur over a few hours and days.

Once the baby has made the transition, in order to maintain effective oxygenation:

- air passages must be clear;
- adequate respiratory exchange must take place in the alveoli;
- circulation must be adequate to transport oxygen to the vital centres;
- the respiratory centre must be active and not suppressed by drugs.

Haemoglobin, which is needed to carry oxygen around the body, is high *in utero* (Stables and Rankin, 2005). After birth this high level is no longer needed and is therefore broken down, which often leads to physiological jaundice in the newborn (this will be discussed further in Chapter 6).

Thermoregulation (temperature maintenance)

One of the key transitions a baby must make is that of maintaining its own temperature (thermoregulation). The fetus has been dependent upon its mother for temperature regulation. In the uterus the fetus has been used to a constant temperature of 37°C (Johnston *et al.*, 2004). Heat has been transferred to the developing fetus via the placenta and the uterus. This results in the fetus having a temperature that is 0.3–0.5°C higher than its mother's (Dede Cinar and Muge Filiz, 2006). Once born the baby must make a number of adjustments. It must become used to maintaining its own temperature in an environment that is significantly cooler that the one it has been used to (the delivery suite temperature is probably around 21–25°C rather than the 37°C the baby has been used to), and get used to a fluctuating temperature rather than one which is constant. The baby is unable to utilise methods used by adults to regulate its temperature and you will be responsible for ensuring that the baby maintains a neutral thermal environment.

Regulation of body temperature

All humans are homoeothermic (warm blooded) (Stables and Rankin, 2005). The maintenance of body temperature in humans depends upon a balance of heat production and heat loss. The hypothalamus in the brain is the major heat regulating centre. It receives input from both thermo receptors in skin and central thermo receptors in the baby's core. The hypothalamus responds to any heat change by initiating heat-promotion or heat-loss mechanisms.

Heat transfer in the body is affected by two gradients. The internal gradient is the transfer from the core of the baby to its surface and the external gradient involves heat transfer from the baby's body surface to the environment (Coad and Dunstall, 2005). The transfer of heat through the internal gradient depends upon insulation and blood flow. Heat loss across the external gradient depends upon the temperature difference between the body and its environment (Coad and Dunstall, 2005).

There are a number of factors that cause poor temperature regulation in babies.

- Babies have a high surface area to body mass ratio (about three times the relative surface area of an adult) (Coad and Dunstall, 2005).
- Babies lack subcutaneous fat (only 16 per cent compared with 30 per cent in adults) (Coad and Dunstall, 2005). This means that heat transfer from the baby's core to the skin (the internal gradient) is rapid.
- Mechanisms of heat conservation and generation regulated by the peripheral nervous system are insufficient in the neonate (Okken, 1991).
- The heat regulating centre in the baby's brain is immature (Farrell and Sittlington, 2003).
- The baby has a limited ability to shiver in order to produce heat and is

limited in its ability to generate heat by muscular activity (Stables and Rankin, 2005).
- Oxygen consumption and metabolic rate increase markedly in response to a drop in temperature (Coad and Dunstall, 2005).

Temperature regulation following birth

As we said above, the baby is no longer in a thermo-constant environment. The delivery room temperature is much lower than the one the baby is used to. The baby is unable to utilise adult methods of thermo-regulation. This means that one of the key areas of care the health professional must give to the baby is to maintain its temperature within normal limits. Generally a newborn baby's rectal temperature may be about 36–37.2°C and its skin temperature between 35.5–36.5°C (Stables and Rankin, 2005).

Perhaps the most important considerations for you as health care professionals caring for newborn babies are the heat loss mechanisms in babies. If you understand these four key mechanisms you will understand the importance of the care you will need to give at birth to help maintain the baby's temperature within normal limits.

Information box 1

Heat loss mechanisms
- **Evaporation** – evaporative heat loss is perhaps the most significant for the newborn baby. Heat loss by evaporation occurs when the skin is wet. When the baby is born the skin is wet with amniotic fluid and the moisture quickly evaporates from the skin surface, taking with it a large amount of heat from the baby (Resuscitation Council UK, 2006). This is why it is so important to dry the baby and replace the wet towel with a new dry towel as soon as possible after delivery.
- **Convection** – convective heat loss is caused by draughts passing by the baby. This means it is important to shut doors and windows and to turn off any fans prior to the baby being born.
- **Conduction** – this is heat loss by contact with a cold surface. It is important to ensure that you don't place a baby on a cold surface following delivery and that, before the baby is born, you try to warm the towels that you will use to dry the baby after delivery.
- **Radiation** – this is heat loss to colder surfaces/objects. You should make sure that you don't place a baby close to a cold surface or object.

> **Information box 2**
>
> **Sources of heat production/gain in the baby**
> - Brown fat (brown adipose tissues (BAT)) stores are an extremely important mechanism for heat production in newborn babies. It is estimated that two to seven per cent of the weight of the newborn baby is thought to consist of BAT (Coad and Dunstall, 2005). BAT is mainly located around the kidneys, the mediastinum, around the nape of neck, the scapulae, along the spinal column and around the large blood vessels in the neck (Stables and Rankin, 2005). BAT cells differ from normal fat cells due to the significant heat production that they are capable of making. However, this process requires the baby to utilise extra oxygen and glucose (Stables and Rankin, 2005).
> - Physical activity such as crying and restlessness also generates heat (Stables and Rankin, 2005).

The effect of cold thermal stress on a neonate may be extremely damaging. Allowing a baby to become cold (hypothermic) may reduce the amount of surfactant produced (which may lead to breathing problems) and hypoglycaemia (low blood sugar which will be discussed further in Chapter 8). This is why it is so important that your care of the baby should ensure a transition to extrauterine life that enables the baby to maintain its temperature within normal limits.

Gastro intestinal tract

In utero all the baby's nutrients have come in a predigested form via the placenta. After birth the baby must suck, swallow, digest, absorb, excrete by itself in order to survive. Feeding will be discussed in much further detail in Chapter 5.

In utero all the baby's waste products have also been excreted by the placenta. The baby must now excrete all its waste products. The baby's kidneys are relatively immature and their ability to concentrate urine is inefficient. Initially the baby will only pass between 15–60 mls of urine per day (Cavaliere, 2003). This will increase to about 200 ml per day for a breastfed baby by the tenth day (Johnston *et al.*, 2004). You would normally expect the baby to have their bowels open within 24 hours (Johnston *et al.*, 2004). These will both be discussed further in Chapter 6.

PREPARATION FOR DELIVERY

As a health care practitioner it is your responsibility to support the baby in making a safe and effective transition to extrauterine life. In order to do this you will need to prepare for the delivery. Most babies make a very effective transition to extrauterine life. However, simple measures will help the baby make an effective change without adverse consequences.

You will need to check the resuscitaire and it is important that you become familiar with the way in which the resuscitaire in your own Hospital Trust works so that, in an emergency, you are able to operate it effectively. Checking resuscitaires thoroughly every day and before each delivery will ensure that you are familiar with both how it works and the equipment that should be on it.

When a delivery is imminent it is important that you close all the doors and windows and switch off any fans (this will help to prevent the baby losing heat by convection). You should ensure that the room is warm and switch on the radiant heater on the resuscitaire. This means that if it is needed the baby will be placed onto a pre-warmed towel, which will help to prevent heat loss by conduction. There should be two towels on the resuscitaire so that the first towel may be discarded once the baby has been dried (Resuscitation Council UK, 2006); this will help prevent heat loss by evaporation. Babies with congenital conditions such as gastraschisis or exomphalus shouldn't be put under a radiant heater as the heater would dry out the exposed bowel.

You should also review the mother's notes and intrapartum history and decide if you need to have a paediatrician present for the delivery. Most NHS Hospital Trusts have a guideline indicating when a paediatrician should be present for delivery. You should familiarise yourself with this document and call for help if the woman and her baby fall into any of these categories. If you need a paediatrician present at delivery you should explain this to the parents.

FOLLOWING THE BIRTH OF THE BABY

You would anticipate that the baby will give a loud and lusty cry, which, in turn, will activate the physiological changes discussed above. For babies who need further support to initiate respirations see neonatal resuscitation below. The NICE Intrapartum Guidelines (2007) recommend that the Apgar score at one and five minutes should be recorded routinely for all births. The Apgar score is a score devised by Virginia Apgar in 1953 in order to assess the condition of babies at birth. The baby is given a score for each sign (see Information box 3 below). The scores are added together and a score is given out of 10 at one minute, five minutes and ten minutes after delivery.

If the baby is born in poor condition (the Apgar score at one minute is 5 or less), then the time to the onset of regular respirations should be recorded and the cord double-clamped to allow paired cord blood gases to be taken. The Apgar score should be recorded at intervals until the baby's condition is stable (NICE, 2007). The more you observe babies at delivery the better you will become at assessing their Apgar score.

Information box 3

Apgar score

Sign	0	1	2
Heart rate	Absent	Slow – below 100/min	Fast -- above 100/min
Respiratory effort	Absent	Slow – irregular	Good, crying
Muscle tone	Limp	Some flexion of extremities	Active
Reflex irritability	No response	Grimace	Crying, cough
Colour	Blue, pale	Body pink, extremities blue	Completely pink

(Stables and Rankin, 2005)

You need to give care to minimise heat loss and maintain a neutral thermal environment for the baby. You have already prepared the room so that the baby will be born into a warm room with no draughts, thus helping to prevent heat loss by convection. If appropriate, women should be encouraged to have skin-to-skin contact with their baby as soon as possible after birth (NICE, 2007). Some women may want to have their baby delivered onto their chest so that they can commence skin-to-skin care straight after delivery. You should ask the mother her preference prior to delivery. In a study by Finigan and Davies (2004) women who had skin-to-skin contact with their babies after birth described feelings of bonding and getting to know their baby demonstrating the importance of early contact between mothers and their babies.

In order to maintain heat the baby should be dried and the wet towel discarded (to help prevent heat loss by evaporation) (Resuscitation Council, 2006). Babies should then be covered with a warm, dry blanket or towel while maintaining skin-to-skin contact with their mother (NICE, 2007). This will help prevent the baby losing further heat by conduction and convection. Initiation of breastfeeding should be encouraged as soon as possible after the birth, preferably within one hour (NICE, 2007). Studies observing women and their newborn babies suggest that physical contact between them encourages attachment (Johnston *et al.*, 2004).

If the baby looks small, a hat will ensure that he or she doesn't lose too much heat from the head. Avoid putting baby on cold surfaces; when weighing babies you can place a warm towel on the scales and then calibrate the scales so that you still get an accurate weight. This will help prevent the baby losing heat via conduction. Be careful in areas such as theatres where the air is changed regularly; this may lead to draughts that put the baby at increased risk of losing heat by convection. You may need to monitor the baby's temperature more closely to ensure it doesn't become cold.

Separation of a woman and her baby within the first hour of the birth for routine postnatal procedures, for example weighing, should be avoided unless these measures are requested by the woman or are necessary for the immediate care of the baby (NICE, 2007). Head circumference, body temperature and the baby's birth weight should be recorded soon after the first hour of birth (NICE, 2007).

Any examination or treatment of the baby should be undertaken with the consent of and in the presence of the parents. If this is not possible, it should be with their knowledge (NICE, 2007). The examinations that are undertaken after the birth of the baby will be discussed further in Chapter 4.

It is important that you write name bands and apply them to the baby. You should check with the parents that the information that you have on the baby's label is correct. Although rare, there are highly publicised cases of babies being incorrectly labelled and being sent home with the wrong parents. It is important to allow parents time to look at and be with their newborn baby soon after delivery.

Vitamin K

You may have seen or be aware that all maternity units offer all newborn babies an injection of vitamin K following birth. This is to prevent Vitamin K Deficiency Bleeding (previously known as Haemorrhagic Disease of the Newborn or HDN). Vitamin K levels in babies are about 50 per cent of adult levels. This means that the babies' ability to clot efficiently is affected (Coad and Dunstall, 2005). Vitamin K Deficiency Bleeding is caused by a deficiency of clotting factors II, VII, IX, X (Dehil-Jones and Fraser Askin, 2004). These clotting factors are dependent on vitamin K. Vitamin K levels are low in newborn babies because placental transport of the vitamin is low and there is a lack of gut intestinal flora in the baby to synthesise vitamin K (Coad, 2004). The baby's gut becomes colonised with flora once feeding is established. There are three forms of Vitamin K Deficiency Bleeding in the newborn.

- **Early** – this presents within the first 48 hours of life. It is usually associated with babies whose mothers have been on medications such as anticonvulsants or warfarin therapy.
- **Classic** – this usually occurs in babies between the second and sixth day of life.
- **Late** – this occurs between 2 and 12 weeks. It is most frequently associated with prolonged breastfeeding without prophylactic vitamin K or only a small dose of oral vitamin K. However, some of these cases are associated with babies who have gastrointestinal or liver disorders causing fat malabsorption.

(Tucker Blackburn, 2003)

Signs and symptoms of Vitamin K Deficiency Bleeding may include:

- gastrointestinal tract bleeding (melaena (black) stools and/or blood-stained vomit);
- bleeding into the central nervous system;
- epistaxis (nose bleeds);
- unexplained bruising;
- oozing of blood from the cord (umbilicus) or neonatal screening site.

(Hey, 2003; Coad and Dunstall, 2005)

If you suspect a baby may be suffering from Vitamin K Deficiency Bleeding you should refer immediately for medical help.

By administering vitamin K at birth, Vitamin K Deficiency Bleeding may be avoided. However, since a study by Golding *et al.* in 1992, in which a link was made between the administration of intramuscular vitamin K, pethidine and childhood cancer, the administration of vitamin K routinely to all babies has sometimes been controversial and parents' permission should be sought prior to its administration. NICE (2006) recommend that all parents should be offered vitamin K prophylaxis for their baby. They recommend that it should be administered as a single dose of 1 mg intramuscularly as this is the most clinically and cost effective method (NICE, 2006). Oral vitamin K should be offered if parents refuse an intramuscular injection of vitamin K (NICE, 2006). However, parents should be advised that it should be given according to the manufacturer's instructions and multiple doses are required.

As a health practitioner you need to consider the advice you are going to give parents to ensure that they make an 'informed choice'. The Royal College of Midwives Position Paper No. 13b (1999) makes a number of statements in relation to the administration of vitamin K that include the following.

- Midwives should give parents accurate and unbiased information (in the antenatal period) to enable them to make an informed choice.
- The Royal College of Midwives (RCM) does not take a position on the current state of research in regard to the safety of vitamin K administration.
- It is up to parents to decide if and how their child should receive vitamin K.
- Despite the risks associated with breastfeeding this should in no way undermine the promotion of breastfeeding.
- Midwives should be alert to episodes of minor bleeding and prolonged jaundice.

Much of the literature concludes that the risk of cancer link is not proven (Ansell *et al.*, 2004). However, we do know that there is a definite risk of Vitamin K Deficiency Bleeding.

DELIVERIES IN WHICH THE BABY NEEDS RESUSCITATION

As we have said, most babies make a successful transition to extrauterine life without the need for resuscitation. However, some babies will require resuscitation and as a health care professional you will be expected to undertake this. It is beyond the remit of this book to explain the process of neonatal resuscitation in full. The algorithm is outlined in Information box 4 but it is important that you go to the Resuscitation Council website and ensure that you read the information in full (**www.resus.org.uk**). The NICE intrapartum guidelines (2007) recommend that all relevant health care professionals caring for women during birth should attend a neonatal resuscitation course at least once a year. It is important that you are familiar with, and attend, regular neonatal resuscitation updates. The guidelines go on to say that the resuscitation session should be consistent with the algorithm adopted in the 'Newborn life support course' developed by the Resuscitation Council (UK) (NICE, 2007).

Information box 4

Resuscitation Algorithm (Resuscitation Council UK, 2006):

Dry the baby

↓

Remove the wet towel and cover the baby with a dry towel.
Start the clock and make a note of the time.

↓

Assess the baby's colour, tone, heart rate and breathing.

↓

If the baby isn't breathing open the airway -- placing the baby's head in a neutral position.

↓

If the baby is still not breathing give five inflation breaths either with an ambu bag or T-piece and face mask.

↓

If there has been no response you should recheck the head position, apply a jaw thrust and repeat the inflation breaths. You should check to see if there is an increase in the baby's heart rate. If there isn't, check chest movement.

↓

If there is no response you should try alternative airway manoeuvres such as using oropharyngeal airway and oral suction and then repeat the inflation breaths. Again you should check to see if there is any increase in heart rate and, if there isn't, check chest movement.

↓

When chest is moving with inflation breaths you can go on to give ventilation breaths. Recheck the heart rate. If the heart rate isn't detectable, or is slow (less than 60) and not increasing you will need to start chest compressions at a rate of three compressions to each breath.

↓

Reassess the baby's heart rate every 30 seconds.
Consider venous access and drugs.

- **Inflation breaths** are breaths given via an ambu bag or T-piece of 2–3 seconds' duration, at 30 cm of water for a term baby.
- **Ventilation breaths** are breaths given via an ambu bag or T-piece and are shorter breaths given at a rate of about 30 per minute.

Basic resuscitation of newborn babies should be started with air (NICE, 2007). Oxygen should be available for any baby that does not respond once adequate ventilation has been established (NICE, 2007).

Most babies will make a safe transition to extrauterine life with minimal support from you. However, you will need to remember that there are things you can do to ensure that the baby doesn't suffer any adverse consequences from the transition. These include ensuring good temperature control and preparing for the delivery so that help and equipment are available if needed.

Key points
- Most babies make an effective transition to extrauterine life with minimal help. As the health care professional involved in this transition you can take important steps to make the transition as smooth as possible for the baby and their parents.
- Health care professionals should prepare for any delivery to ensure that all equipment is in good working order and that measures are undertaken to minimise heat loss to the newborn baby.
- Health care professionals should be aware of the current information in relation to vitamin K administration and consider what information they should give to parents.
- Health care professionals should undertake regular updates in neonatal resuscitation and be aware of the guidance given on neonatal resuscitation by the Resuscitation Council UK.

Exercises

1. You are caring for Julie who is at 40 weeks' gestation and is in the second stage of labour. Your mentor thinks that the delivery will be in the next 15 minutes. What preparations do you need to make for the delivery and why?
2. Baby Tara is one hour old and you need to ask her parents for consent to administer a vitamin K injection. What information/explanation would you give them?
3. Baby Zac has just been born but makes little breathing effort when he is born. What will you need to do and why?

REFERENCES

Ansell, P., Roman, E., Fear, N., Simpson, J., Day, N. and Eden, T. (2004) 'Vitamin K update: survey of paediatricians in the UK'. *British Journal of Midwifery* 12 (1): 38–41

Cavaliere, T. (2003) 'Genitourinary Assessment', in Taperro, E. and Honeyfield, M.E. (2003) *Physical Assessment of the Newborn: A*

Comprehensive Approach to the Art of Physical Examination (3rd Ed.). Santa Rosa, CA: NICU INK

Coad, J. with Dunstall, M. (2005) *Anatomy and Physiology for Midwives* (2nd Ed). Edinburgh: Elsevier Churchill Livingstone

Dede Cinar, N. and Muge Filiz, T. (2006) 'Neonatal thermoregulation'. *Journal of Neonatal Nursing*, 12: 69–74

Dehil-Jones, W. and Fraser Askin, D. (2004) 'Hematologic Disorders', in Verklan, T. and Walden, M. (2004) *Core Curriculum for Neonatal Intensive Care Nursing*. Philadelphia: Elsevier Saunders

Farrell, P. and Sittlington, N. (2003) 'The Normal Baby' in Fraser, D. and Cooper, M., (2003) *Myles Textbook for Midwives* (14th Ed.). Edinburgh: Churchill Livingstone

Finigan, V. and Davies, S. (2004) ' "I just wanted to love, hold him forever": women's lived experience of skin to skin contact with their baby immediately after birth'. *Evidence Based Midwifery*, 2 (2): 59–65

Fraser Askin, D. (2002) 'Complications in the Transition From Fetal to Neonatal Life'. *Journal of Obstetric, Gynecologic, and Neonatal Nursing*, 31 (3): 318–326

Fraser, D. (2003) 'Chest and Lungs Assessment', in Taperro, E. and Honeyfield, M.E. *Physical Assessment of the Newborn: A Comprehensive approach to the Art of Physical Examination* (3rd Ed.). Santa Rosa, CA: NICU INK

Golding, J., Greenwood, R., Birmingham, K. and Mott, M. (1992) 'Childhood cancer, intramuscular vitamin K, and pethidine given during labour'. *British Medical Journal*, 305: 341–346

Hey, E. (2003) 'Vitamin K – what, why, and when'. *Arch Dis Child Fetal Neonatal Ed*, 88: F80–83

Johnston, P., Flood, K. and Spinks, K. (2004) *The Newborn Child* (9th Ed.). Edinburgh: Churchill Livingstone

National Institute for Health and Clinical Excellence (2006) *Routine postnatal care of women and their babies*. London: NICE

National Institute for Health and Clinical Excellence (2007) *Intrapartum Guidelines*. London: NICE

Okken, A. (1991) 'Postnatal adaptation in thermoregulation'. *Journal of Perinatal Medicine*, 19 (Supp 1): 67–73

Resuscitation Council UK (2006) *Newborn Life Support Resuscitation at Birth* (2nd Ed). London: Resuscitation Council (UK)

Royal College of Midwives (1999) Position Paper No. 13 b, Vitamin K. *RCM Midwives Journal*, 2: 252–3

Stables, D. and Rankin, J. (2005) *Physiology in Childbearing with Anatomy and Related Biosciences* (2nd Ed.). London: Elsevier

Tucker Blackburn, S. (2003) *Maternal, Fetal and Neonatal Physiology* (2nd Ed.). Philadelphia: W.B. Saunders

Useful Websites

Resuscitation Council guidelines

www.resus.org.uk

Chapter 4

Neonatal Screening
Cathy Coppinger

Chapter aims

To explore neonatal newborn screening, the role of the nurse or midwife and the significance of findings.

Learning outcomes
By the end of this chapter you will be able to:
- demonstrate an understanding of the screening of neonates, including the midwife's initial birth examination, the medical neonatal examination, neonatal hearing screening and newborn blood spot screening;
- discuss the midwife's and nurse's role in the screening processes and the significance of findings.

Mapping to standards of proficiency

Standards of Proficiency for Pre-registration Midwifery Education (SPME)
Effective Midwifery Practice
Examine and care for babies immediately following birth. This will include:
- confirming their vital signs and taking the appropriate action;
- full assessment and physical examination.

Examine and care for babies with specific health or social needs and refer to other professionals or agencies as appropriate. This will include:
- congenital disorders;
- birth defects.

Standards of Proficiency for Pre-registration Nursing Education
Collaborate with patients and clients and, when appropriate, additional carers to review and monitor the progress of individuals or groups towards planned outcomes.

INTRODUCTION

This chapter will discuss neonatal newborn screening, the role of the nurse or midwife and the significance of findings. All parents in the UK are offered screening for their babies. Newborn screening includes the newborn physical examination (sometimes known as the 'medical examination'), hearing and blood spot screening. The initial examination of the baby soon after birth by a midwife, although not a screening procedure, is included in this chapter. Each region in England and all UK countries have antenatal and newborn screening teams. The core remit of regional teams is the implementation and monitoring of appropriate antenatal and newborn screening and the provision of appropriate education, and training is key to this (Harcombe, 2007).

Raffle and Gray (2007, p. 37) define screening as 'the testing of people without signs or symptoms of the condition being tested for, with the purpose of reducing the risk of ill health in relation to the condition being tested, or giving them information about the risk'. Screening tests are never 100 per cent sensitive. Babies with an abnormal screening result may turn out not to have the condition for which they are tested (which is known as a 'false positive'). Nor are screening tests 100 per cent specific and some babies affected by the condition can be missed (this is known as a 'false negative') (DH, 2007). It is important that the health care practitioner is aware that false positives and false negatives may occur in screening so that they remain vigilant for signs of diseases that may not have been picked up in the screening process.

Babies who are thought to be at higher risk of a condition are referred on for further tests and a definitive diagnosis. Appropriate diagnostic and treatment services must be in place for babies who screen positive (Raffle and Gray, 2007). Reports of delay in the initiation of treatment are widespread (Knowles *et al.*, 2005; Rahi and Dezateux, 1999); protocols must ensure timely access to the appropriate specialist and the health care professional must be familiar with all the steps in the screening programme so that timely and appropriate referrals can be made.

The National Screening Committee (NSC) set criteria for appraising the viability, effectiveness and appropriateness of a screening programme. In summary, the condition must be an important health problem where early identification and treatment, before symptoms develop, can reduce severity. There must be an acceptable screening test available that performs well. The benefit from the screening programme should outweigh the physical and psychological harm (caused by the test, diagnostic procedures and treatment) and it must be cost-effective (NSC, 2003).

Although screening is focused on the detection of abnormality, it is accepted that newborn physical examination has a more holistic function of confirming health and normality and providing education for parents in terms of their baby's physiology, abilities and needs (NHS QIS, 2004; Hall and Elliman, 2004; NICE, 2006).

CONSENT

Informed choice is a central part of health care policy in the UK (NICE, 2003; DH 2004; UK Newborn Screen Programme Centre (UKNSPC), 2005) and is essential in gaining consent (DH, 2001; Clinical Negligence Scheme for Trusts (CNST), 2004). The health care practitioner is responsible for gaining consent prior to performing the screening procedures and must be able to communicate clearly with the baby's parents. This will include sharing evidence-based information on the purpose, procedure, accessing results, possible findings and treatment options. Although newborn screening tests are recommended, parents have the choice to accept or decline screening. For further information on obtaining consent see Chapter 10.

All information for parents should be in a form that is accessible, taking into account any additional needs such as physical, cognitive or sensory disabilities and people who do not speak or read English (NICE, 2006). It should be provided in the antenatal period and immediately before the test (Stewart *et al.*, 2004). The NSC has produced a parents' information booklet 'Screening tests for you and your baby' to assist parents in their decision to accept or decline screening for their baby. The parents' decision should be recorded in the maternity/baby records and in the 'Personal Child Health Record' (PCHR), the main record of a child's health, growth and development. The health care practitioner will be responsible for ensuring that a valid consent is obtained and that it has been documented.

THE INITIAL AND NEWBORN PHYSICAL EXAMINATION

The initial examination of the baby is usually undertaken by the midwife shortly after birth. Although it isn't classed as a screening procedure it is included within this chapter as there is overlap between the initial midwifery examination and the newborn physical (medical) examination. The newborn physical examination is a more detailed examination that includes examination of heart, hips and eyes, and these components will be discussed in more detail below. The newborn physical examination is undertaken by medical staff or by advanced neonatal nurse practitioners, midwives or neonatal nurses who have undertaken further specialist training to enable them to carry out the physical examination of the newborn.

The initial examination marks the beginning of child health surveillance; however, it includes consideration of the antenatal period, including a review of any results of screening for infection, congenital abnormalities, fetal anomaly and growth monitoring. Fetal anomaly scans detect about half of the major abnormalities that can cause serious difficulties (RCOG, 2000). Both examinations involve a review of the family, antenatal and perinatal history and a top-to-toe assessment of a baby that is thought to be well and nursed on a postnatal ward or at home. They also provide opportunity for health promotion (NHS QIS, 2004; NICE, 2006).

Initial examination

To encourage the initiation of breastfeeding, separation of a woman and her baby should be avoided within the first hour after birth (NICE, 2006). The initial examination should be performed soon after, with the mother's consent and, where possible, with the mother and father present (DH, 2004; NICE, 2006). The aim of the initial examination is to reassure parents that their baby appears normal and to detect any major physical abnormality or problems that require referral (Baston and Durward, 2001; Hall and Elliman, 2004). The health care practitioner should ensure that the environment is light, so that they can inspect the baby clearly; and warm, to ensure that the baby doesn't become cold during the examination (see Chapter 3 on temperature control). The examinations should be undertaken in private whenever possible as confidential information may be discussed. Hands should be washed and dried to prevent any cross-infection. Any equipment to be used should be clean and correctly functioning. The health care practitioner should not undertake the initial assessment of a baby until they have first observed the midwife carrying out the examination and been observed undertaking the examination with their mentor or assessor.

The health care practitioner will need to ask the mother information about her baby's behaviour and activities of feeding, elimination and sleep patterns. The health care practitioner must also absorb information from the baby's responses and behaviour through senses of sight, touch and hearing. Most of the information needed for a complete physical assessment can be gained solely through observation (Tappero and Honeyfield, 2003). The baby should be handled respectfully, only those parts being examined should be exposed, the examination should be explained, permission sought and the baby comforted as required. The more the health care practitioner observes and examines babies the better they will become at detecting when the baby is unwell or needs further support.

The baby's head circumference, body temperature and birth weight are measured and recorded during the examination (NICE, 2007).

The head

The health care practitioner will need to gently palpate the skull, the sutures and the anterior and posterior fontanelles, which are normally open and soft. Skull bones may overlap due to moulding. This is quite normal and parents should be reassured that this is so and that their baby's head will return to a normal shape in a few days.

Caput succedaneum is a swelling caused by pressure during birth and this may be visible. Caput succedaneum is a common feature caused by oedema (swelling) of the newborn scalp; the swelling may cross the suture lines. Again parents should be reassured that this will settle down in a few days. Undue pressure on the fetal head during birth may also cause cephalhaematoma. Cephalhaematoma is caused by bleeding below the periosteum (the skull bone), resulting in swelling. This swelling is assigned to separate skull bones and does not cross suture lines (Johnson, 1994, cited in Kanneh and Davies, 2000). These swellings can be alarming to parents and the examiner must explain the cause, care of the scalp, and reassure parents that the conditions will resolve spontaneously in six to eight weeks.

The head circumference is measured midway between the hairline and the eyebrows and the occipital prominence (back of head). In a term baby the average is 35–36 cm (Kanneh and Davies, 2000). It is recorded in maternity notes and plotted on the centile chart in the PCHR (Child Growth Foundation and Royal College of Paediatrics and Child Health, 2004).

The ears should be positioned at the level of an extended line from inner to outer canthus (the angle at either end of the eye) (Tappero and Honeyfield, 2003). The cartilage in the ear should be well developed in a term baby.

The face

The face should look symmetrical. The normal baby has two eyes. The inner and outer canthi (the edges of the eyes) should be level. The eye opening is called the palpebral fissure and the distance between the inner canthus of the eyes is the length of one palpebral fissure (Tappero and Honeyfield, 2003). The eyes should be clear, the iris is coloured dark grey or blue and the sclera white. The eyes can become bruised and oedematous (swollen) due to birth trauma, and conjunctival haemorrhage (bleeding) may be seen.

The nose should be placed vertically in the midline and the nostrils should be patent. The colour of the lips and membranes should be pink. The health care practitioner will need to check that the hard and soft palate inside the baby's mouth is intact. The sucking and gag reflexes are usually noted during palpation of the hard and soft palate. The health care practitioner can check the palates by gently inserting a clean finger inside the baby's mouth and checking that the roof of the baby's mouth is intact. If they insert their finger gently further back then the health care practitioner may check for the soft palate.

The skin

The skin is normally clear, soft and elastic. Vernix caseosa, a greasy white material that covers the baby's skin, may be present but the amount decreases as the baby reaches term. Lanugo, a soft downy hair, may be present but this also lessens towards term. The skin colour should be normal for ethnicity (NICE, 2006). The health care practitioner needs to become used to observing babies of different ethnic origins so that they become familiar with a baby's 'normal' colour. However, all babies should be centrally pink. A good place to check this is the lips, which should be pink. The baby may have acrocyanosis, where the hands and feet look slightly cyanosed (a blue discolouration). This is normal and usually resolves after 24 hours. Cyanosis (blueness) other than acrocyanosis, or jaundice (see Chapters 6 and 8) in the first few hours of life always needs referral to medical aid and investigation.

Posture and movement

The baby should be in an attitude of flexion. The limbs should be equal in length and the legs flexed and abducted, lying away from the midline of the body; the arms flexed and adducted, lying towards the midline of the body. Five separate fingers and toes should be counted on each hand and foot respectively. The nails in a term baby should be formed and there should be creases on the hand palm and the soles of the feet. When the baby moves its limbs the movement should be symmetrical with good muscle tone. The baby's feet should be straight, in a neutral position with good range of movement. The midwife will also see if the baby has normal reflexes (see Information box 1).

Information box 1

Normal reflexes
- Sucking reflex.
- Gagging reflex.
- Grasp reflex, where the baby curls its fingers around the examiner's finger.
- Babinski reflex, where the big toe flexes and the toes fan out in response to stroking the plantar (middle of foot) region.
- Moro reflex, also known as the startle reflex, where in response to a feeling of falling, both arms are abducted with fingers wide open followed by adduction.
- Stepping reflex. When the baby is held upright and its feet touch a hard, flat surface, the baby will make stepping movements.

The chest and abdomen

The chest should be symmetrical (equal) and breast and nipple tissue developed in a term baby. The clavicles are observed and palpated for any fractures that may have occurred during delivery. Normal respirations are symmetrical (equal) and diaphragmatic (chest); the rate should be 30–60 breaths per minute. The normal heart rate is 120–160 beats per minute (NICE, 2006). The temperature should be taken in the axilla (under the arm) using a digital thermometer. Normal body temperature in a normal room environment (20°C) is around 37°C (NICE, 2006).

Genitalia

The health care practitioner examines the genitalia to ensure the baby has a normal urethral opening and passage of urine. Ninety-eight per cent of term babies will pass urine in the first 30 hours of life (Tappero and Honeyfield, 2003). Patency of the anus is confirmed by the passage of meconium, which normally occurs in the first 12–24 hours (Kanneh and Davies, 2000).

The back

The spine should be flat and the vertebral column (back bones) straight. The skin on the baby's back should be clear with no sacral dimples or tufts of hair. Mongolian blue spots (a blue area at the base of the spine that may look like a bruise) is a normal finding in some ethnic groups. Leg length and symmetry of creases may be examined while baby is in the prone (lying on its tummy) position.

The baby should be weighed naked using a digital scale which is regularly calibrated and placed on a firm surface (Hall and Elliman, 2004). Average weight in a term baby is approximately 3.5 kg. The abdomen should appear symmetrical and the umbilical cord clamp should be checked to make sure it is secure.

If the health care practitioner knows the normal physical characteristics of a healthy term baby they are then able to identify differences and abnormal features that may need further investigation. For example, recognisable features for a baby with Down's Syndrome may include upslanted eyes, flat occiput (back of head) and small white flecks seen in the iris, called Brushfield spots. The limbs and fingers can be slightly shorter than average with a single palmar crease. The toes may have a gap between the first and second toe known as a sandal gap. Muscle tone is usually poor at birth and congenital heart defects are much more common (Fetal Anomaly Screening Programme (FASP), 2007).

Dysmorphic (abnormal) features are found in babies with chromosomal abnormalities but can also be seen in babies with no problems. Other examples of features that may indicate a problem are a large or small head circumference where abnormal brain/skull growth has occurred.

Once it is completed, the health care practitioner should record the initial examination in the maternity/baby records, and birth details, weight and measurements are recorded in the PCHR. Feeding patterns and elimination of urine and meconium are also recorded. If abnormal features are detected the baby should be referred to a paediatrician or other health professional with the necessary skills and experience.

Newborn physical examination

The newborn physical examination is a more thorough physical examination of the newborn performed within 72 hours of birth. The newborn physical examination comprises the elements above but also includes screening for congenital cardiac defects, developmental dysplasia of the hip, some eye disorders (including congenital cataract), and undescended testes in males (NHS QIS, 2004; NICE, 2006). This examination is repeated at 6–8 weeks of age. As said above, the examination is either undertaken by a doctor or by a health care practitioner who has undertaken further training in this area.

Screening for congenital heart defects

The examiner will observe the baby but will also listen to the heart and lungs with a stethoscope. Congenital heart defects affect 7–8 per 1 000 live births. Screening aims to identify life-threatening congenital heart defects before symptoms arise, to achieve timely diagnosis, described as preoperative diagnosis before collapse or death occurs. A secondary objective is the detection of clinically significant congenital heart defects (Knowles *et al.*, 2005). About 25 per cent of congenital heart defects are detected on fetal anomaly scans (RCOG, 2000) and examination of newborn babies detects less than half of those with congenital cardiac malformation (Ainsworth *et al.*, 1999). The examination takes place at a time of rapid change within the cardiovascular system as part of adaptation to extrauterine life, so it may be difficult for the examiner to detect the abnormality. This means that the health care practitioner with continuing care for the baby will need to continue to observe the baby for further signs of a congenital heart condition (such as cyanosis – blueness) that may be seen in the baby later.

Information box 2

Risk factors for a congenital heart condition
- Down's syndrome, where 35–40 per cent have cardiovascular malformations (Ainsworth *et al.* 1999).
- Family history of a congenital heart condition (Park, 2002).
- Antenatal infections such as rubella increase the risk of a congenital heart condition.

For the clinical examination the baby is undressed and is examined in a calm state. Clinical examination involves observation of activity, tone and skin colour. An assessment of heart rate, rhythm, regularity and the presence of abnormal heart sounds or murmurs is made by the examiner with a stethoscope. Respirations (breathing) are also assessed with the examiner moving from top to bottom and systematically side to side. The lower lobes of the lungs are assessed through the baby's back. The chest should normally be quiet.

All babies who screen positively need further evaluation by a more experienced examiner such as a specialist paediatric registrar or consultant neonatologist or paediatrician. Pulse oximetry may be undertaken to assist diagnosis. Pulse oximetry identifies hypoxaemia (low oxygen) in the blood. Pulse oximetry as a screening test for congenital heart disease in newborn babies is currently being evaluated (**www.hta.ac.uk/**

1624NIHR Health Technology Assessment Programme). Following further examination by the experienced examiner the baby may be referred for a detailed diagnostic echocardiogram. This allows the four chambers of the heart, the large blood vessels and the heart valves to be seen while the heart is beating, but may not be available immediately.

Congenital cataracts

Screening for congenital cataracts and other eye abnormalities is part of the newborn physical examination (NSC, 2006a; NSC, 2005). The implications for the baby if the defect is not detected is impairment of vision and potential blindness (Rahi and Dezateux, 1999). There are critical periods in normal eye development. The brain relies on clear images to develop its visual pathway, and visual impairments may cause an irreversible reduction in visual perception known as amblyopia (NSC, 2005). The aims of screening are to prevent blindness due to amblyopia. There are two to three cases of congenital cataract per 10000 births, of which one third or less is unilateral (NSC, 2005). The physical newborn examination detects less than half of cases (Rahi and Dezateux, 1999).

Information box 3

Risk factors for congenital cataracts
- Infections such as rubella, toxoplasmosis varicella, cytomegalovirus or herpes.
- Links with genetic syndrome such as, for example, Turner's syndrome.
- Links with metabolic disorders such as galactosaemia.

(Robins, 2001)

Examining the eyes is not always easy as the newborn baby sleeps for long periods and their eyes may be swollen or bruised. Changing the baby's position, as well as gentle to and fro rocking, can sometimes encourage the baby to open his or her eyes. The examination includes observation of the general appearance of the eyes for normal position, shape, symmetry; and observation for any abnormal eye movements, response and behaviour. The eyes are inspected with an ophthalmoscope to ensure the baby has a red reflex. The red reflex is a reflection of a clear red colour from the retina when a bright light is directed at the newborn lens (Tappero and Honeyfield, 2003). The ophthalmoscope is held close to the eye and the examiner looks along the light beam, which is directed into the baby's pupils from a distance of about 15 centimetres. Failure to see the red reflex and a cloudy cornea suggest a cataract and signs of posterior eye disease such as, for example, retinoblastoma. These are indications for urgent referral to an ophthalmologist, preferably a paediatric specialist (NSC, 2005). Congenital cataract is treated by surgically removing the affected lens. Early surgery leads to a good outcome. Treatment is recommended before the age of three months (Rahi and Dezateux, 1999).

Developmental Dysplasia of the Hip (DDH)

This term refers to a range of hip disorders that includes part or complete dislocation of the femoral head from the acetabulum and acetabular dysplasia with or without displacement (Elbourne *et al.*, 2002). The national screening programme introduced in 1969 uses the Ortolani–Barlow test. This test aims to identify infants with hip instability who are at increased risk of hip displacement, in order to stabilise the hip with abduction therapy (NSC, 2004). Dezateux *et al.* (2003) describe a subsidiary goal, which is to achieve this outcome without recourse to surgery. It is believed that early treatment reduces the need for surgery and minimises the long-term disability due to early degenerative joint disease that is associated with the disorder (NSC, 2004). There is a wide range in incidence reported and it is likely that this is due to variation in case definition, variation in screening and diagnostic measures in addition to ethnic and geographic factors (Witt, 2003; Dezateux *et al.*, 2003). The NSC (2004) reports the incidence as 1.2/1 000 births. The incidence is further confused because many hips that are unstable in the newborn period spontaneously resolve in the first two weeks after birth (Witt, 2003).

Information box 4

Risk factors for DDH
- Family history.
- Breech presentation.
- Primiparity (first baby).
- Oligohydramnios (small amount of amniotic fluid surrounding the baby).
- Female sex (Chan *et al.*, 1997; Goss, 2002; Elbourne, *et al.*, 2002).
- Talipes, myelomeningocele and other neuromuscular disorders are associated with the disorder (Witt, 2003).

Current guidelines recommend that the Ortolani and Barlow tests be performed within 48 hours of age and at six to eight weeks. In order for the tests to be reliable the baby must be warm and comfortable and there should be little or ideally no resistance. The baby should be lying on a flat surface, in the supine position (on its back) with their nappy off (Jones, 1998; Townsend *et al.*, 2004). The examination includes an assessment of the baby's posture, position, discomfort from bone or joint movement, range of joint motion, muscle size, symmetry, strength and the configuration and motility of the back (Tappero and Honeyfield, 2003). In the Ortolani test the contra lateral hip is held still while the hip being tested is abducted and gently pulled anteriorly. The sensation of instability in a positive Ortolani test is the palpable and sometimes audible 'clunk' as the femoral head moves over a poorly developed posterior rim of the acetabulum and relocating into the cavity (French *et al.*, 1999). Restriction of abduction may indicate an irreducible dislocation (Jones, 1998).

The Barlow test is performed by adducting the hip while pushing the thigh posteriorly. A positive Barlow test is a palpable clunk as the hip goes out of the socket; the hip is dislocatable (French *et al.*, 1999; Jones, 1998). Babies who screen positive should be referred to an orthopaedic surgeon. The NSC advocates clinical screening with selective ultrasound for infants with risk factors or clinical signs present. Ultrasound is not currently recommended for primary screening (NSC, 2004). Early treatment usually consists of abduction splinting.

Cryptochordism (undescended testes)

Early diagnosis and management of the undescended testicle are needed to preserve fertility and improve early detection of testicular malignancy (NSC, 2006b). The incidence of cryptochordism (undescended testes) present at birth is approximately three per cent in term infants (higher in preterm infants) with spontaneous descent occurring in two thirds of cases by age three to six months (Kelsberg *et al.*, 2006).

Information box 5

Risk factors of cryptochordism
- Oligohydramnios (too little amniotic fluid).
- Polyhydramnios (too much amniotic fluid).

(Tappero and Honeyfield, 2003)

By term the testes should be well situated in the scrotum. When palpated, normal testes are firm and smooth and equal in size. They are ovoid in shape, usually mobile and measure on average 1.4 to 1.6 mm in the term neonate (Tappero and Honeyfield, 2003). The genitalia are examined for evidence of hypospadias or ambiguity. Failure to palpate the testes in the scrotum is indication for referral to a paediatric urologist. Treatment may be hormonal or surgical (Kelsberg *et al.*, 2006).

The health care practitioner needs to be aware of the features of the initial examination as well as the more detailed physical examination of the newborn. This will enable them both to undertake the initial examination and also to advise and support parents when their baby has a physical newborn examination, particularly if an abnormality is detected.

Newborn hearing screening

Newborn hearing screening is undertaken to enable detection of bilateral, permanent hearing impairment. Newborn hearing screening results in early diagnosis and treatment of hearing loss. This leads to better outcomes for children and their families in terms of speech, language and social development (Davis *et al.*, 1997). The estimated prevalence is one to two per 1 000 in well babies. The estimated prevalence increases in babies with risk factors for hearing loss and is 10–20 times higher in Neonatal Intensive Care Unit or Special Care Baby Unit populations. There are two models for the screening programme: a hospital-based model using dedicated screeners who offer the test prior to discharge; and a community-based model offered by health visitors.

> **Information box 6**
>
> **Risk factors for hearing impairment**
> - Family history of hearing problems.
> - Prematurity.
> - Craniofacial anomalies.
> - Infection.

The hearing programme tests babies' hearing using an Automated Otoacoustic Emissions test (AOAE). It works on the principle that a healthy cochlear will produce a faint echo when stimulated with a sound. A small earpiece containing a speaker and a microphone is placed in the baby's ear. A clicking sound is played and if the ear is functioning properly the earpiece will pick up the echo and this is recorded on a computer. This test checks if sound is being sent from the cochlear through the auditory nerve to the brain. No further tests are needed if a clear response is heard in both ears. It can be difficult to get a clear response if the baby is unsettled, the room is noisy or if there is fluid in the ear from birth. A second test, known as the Automated Auditory Brainstem Response (AABR) test is offered if the AOAE test does not show a strong response in one or both ears. Soft lightweight headphones are placed on the baby's ears and sensors placed on the baby's head. A series of sounds is played at different levels of loudness and frequencies. The sensors pick up information about the signals that pass along the auditory nerve and send information to the computer, which is interpreted by an audiologist ((National Deaf Children's Society) NDCS, 2005).

Babies who do not show strong responses to either the AOAE or AABR tests are referred to the local audiology department for further tests. The screening process should be complete by five weeks of age (NICE, 2006) but ongoing observation of the baby is encouraged and parents are given checklists for the sounds that babies should make and react to as they get older.

Earlier diagnosis of permanent childhood hearing impairment enables earlier intervention, which is generally agreed to lead to better outcomes, whether through family support, communication support or specific technology-based interventions such as hearing aids or cochlear implants.

Newborn blood spot screening

Newborn blood spot screening identifies babies who may have rare but serious conditions. The NSC recommend that all babies in the UK are offered screening for phenylketonuria (PKU), congenital hypothyroidism (CHT), sickle cell disease (SCD), cystic fibrosis (CF) and medium chain acyl-CoA dehydrogenase deficiency (MCADD).

Newborn blood spot screening tests are performed on dried blood spot specimens collected on a specially designed blood spot card. The blood is collected from the baby's heel between five to eight days after birth, ideally on day five (counting the date of birth as day 0). Usually the health care practitioner who is caring for the baby on day five is responsible for ensuring that the newborn blood spot screening is undertaken appropriately and sent off. The health care practitioner will be responsible for obtaining informed consent to undertake the screening test and will need to have an understanding of the conditions being screened for. The health care practitioner should not undertake the newborn blood spot screening test until they have been trained appropriately.

> **Information box 7**
>
> **Newborn blood spot screening**
> Newborn blood spot screening is normally carried out when baby is five to eight days old. This test screens for the following:
>
> - phenylketonuria (PKU);
> - congenital hypothyroidism (CHT);
> - cystic fibrosis (CF);
> - sickle cell disease (SCD); and
> - medium chain acyl-CoA dehydrogenase deficiency (MCADD).

Phenylketonuria (PKU)

PKU has an incidence of one in 10 000 babies. PKU is an autosomal recessive genetic condition, which means that affected babies have inherited one copy of the altered gene that causes PKU from their mother and one from their father. If a person has only one copy of the altered gene that causes PKU, they are a healthy carrier of the condition (UKNSPC, 2005).

PKU is caused by a deficiency of a liver enzyme called phenylalanine hydroxylase, which is necessary to break down phenylalanine, an amino acid present in many foods. This enzyme is needed to convert phenylalanine into tyrosine, which is essential for normal brain development after birth. People with PKU accumulate too much phenylalanine in the body and not enough tyrosine. The high blood phenylalanine is measured by the laboratory to detect PKU. If left untreated it almost always leads to severe mental disability as well as seizures. In patients with PKU who are not treated, delayed development usually first becomes noticeable between six and 12 months of age, by which time up to 50 IQ points will have been lost (Seymour et al., 1997). Effective therapy to lower raised blood phenylalanine levels by dietary restriction of phenylalanine prevents progressive, irreversible cognitive damage but does not reverse pre-existing damage, and so the earlier that treatment is commenced the better the ultimate outcome (Pollitt et al., 1997). Babies who screen positive for PKU should be referred for treatment by 21 days of age (UKNSPC, 2005).

It is possible for mothers to breastfeed their babies with PKU so long as they balance the amount of breast milk with the baby's special dietary supplement. This may require mothers to express and discard their breast milk initially, until their baby's phenylalanine levels are within target levels (UKNSPC, 2005).

Congenital hypothyroidism (CHT)

CHT has an incidence of one in 4 000 babies and is more common in girls than boys, with a ratio of 2.3 girls to every one boy (UKNSPC, 2005). The majority of cases of CHT are sporadic with a low risk of recurrence in subsequent pregnancies.

In CHT the thyroid gland fails to function normally and a deficiency of the hormone thyroxine results. Primary hypothyroidism is caused by a defect of the gland as a result of an absence or lack of normal development of the thyroid gland, or by an inborn error of one of the several steps in the production of the principal thyroid hormone, thyroxine. Secondary hypothyroidism is the result of a defect that leads to very low levels, or complete absence, of thyroid stimulating hormone (thyrotropin). The thyroid gland itself is normal (Pollitt *et al.*, 1997). The mother's own thyroid doesn't provide enough thyroxine to maintain sufficiently high levels in the fetus.

Information box 8

Symptoms of CHT
In very severe cases of CHT babies are born with, or quickly develop, the following symptoms:

- a very low hair line;
- a protruding tongue;
- cold skin;
- protruding tummy button;
- jaundice;
- feeding difficulties;
- constipation;
- sluggish behaviour.

(UKNSPC, 2005)

However, only very few babies will have all of the symptoms above and primary CHT is rarely diagnosed by clinical means in the newborn period. Thyroid-stimulating hormone produced by the pituitary gland is raised in CHT and can be detected by the laboratory screening test. Babies who screen positive for CHT should be referred for treatment by 21 days of age (UKNSPC, 2005).

If babies with CHT are not treated, they fail to grow properly and will have 'mild to severe' mental disability. In the most severe cases children also have a lack of co-ordination, jerky movements and tremors. In general, patients with complete absence of the thyroid gland (called thyroid agenesis) are the most severely affected. Treatment is by replacing thyroxine with a dose taken by mouth.

Cystic fibrosis (CF)

Cystic fibrosis is an autosomal recessive genetic condition, affecting one in 2 500 babies. In CF there is a problem transporting chloride across cell membranes. This affects certain organs in the body, particularly the pancreas and lungs. The thick secretions in these organs cause digestive problems and chest infections. The abnormal transport of chloride in sweat glands leads to an increased level of chloride in babies' sweat. This is the basis of the 'sweat test' used to investigate suspected cases.

Cystic fibrosis can affect the baby before birth. Fifteen per cent of affected babies are born with blocked intestines, a condition called meconium ileus. Testing for CF is in two stages. The first test measures immunoreactive trypsinogen (IRT). Specimens with a raised IRT are then tested for common DNA alterations for CF. The gene is called cystic fibrosis transmembrane regulator or CFTR gene. CF is caused by a large number of different alterations on the CFTR gene. UK screening laboratories only test for the most common, which means newborn screening will not identify some babies with rare alterations on the CFTR gene. In addition to identifying risk or providing diagnosis for a disorder, genetic testing can reveal carrier status and possibly non-paternity in autosomal recessive genetic conditions (Raffle and Gray, 2007).

Treatment of children with CF aims to improve nutrition by providing supplements containing enzymes to help digestion, and to reduce chest infections with frequent physiotherapy and either occasional or continuous antibiotics. Treatment can slow down the effects of the disease, but cannot stop it progressing. Studies have demonstrated benefits in nutrition, respiratory function and survival (Rock, 2007; Seymour, 1997; Farrell, 2001). Newborn screening for CF may also reduce any delays in diagnosis, lessening anxiety and uncertainty about why the child is ill. Early diagnosis through screening of a baby with CF can also alert the parents to their risk of having other affected children.

Sickle cell disease (SCD)

Sickle cell diseases are rare autosomal recessive genetic diseases that affect the haemoglobin in the red cells. Incidence is one in 2 400 babies. Sickle cell affects the normal oxygen-carrying capacity and when cells are deoxygenated and under stress they can take on a sickle shape, become stiff and then get stuck in small blood vessels. This means the oxygen in the blood is unable to reach parts of the body. As a result people can experience very severe pain known as a 'crisis'. People with sickle cell often experience complications from the disease such as problems with major organs, damage to joints or even strokes. They are also more vulnerable to infections and may have to take antibiotics during childhood and throughout their lives (UKNSPC, 2005).

If the test comes back positive the management of SCD is based on routine prophylactic penicillin for infants and the early use of antibiotics to prevent overwhelming infection. Babies should have been offered and prescribed antibiotics by the time they are three months old (NHS Sickle and Thalassaemia screening programme, 2006).

Medium chain acyl-CoA dehydrogenase deficiency

Medium chain acyl-CoA dehydrogenase deficiency (MCADD) is a rare autosomal recessive genetic condition affecting one in 10 000–20 000 babies born in the UK (Pollitt, 1997). MCADD occurs when the enzyme called medium chain acyl-CoA dehydrogenase is either missing or not functioning properly. This enzyme breaks down the body's own fat to make energy. Babies affected by MCADD often do not show any symptoms straight after birth. Symptoms typically appear for the first time when a child is between three months and three years old (Pollitt, 1997). This usually happens following a period of fasting or infection, for example if the child feels unwell and does not want to eat or vomits (Grosse *et al.*, 2006).

Information box 9

Symptoms of MCADD
Symptoms of MCADD can be highly variable but may include:

- drowsiness or lethargy;
- diarrhoea;
- vomiting;
- fits;
- the baby may go into a coma (this is called a 'metabolic crisis').

MCADD is tested by measuring octanoyl carnitine levels in the blood. Babies who screen positive should be referred to a specialist metabolic paediatrician. If MCADD is not identified early, children affected by the disorder may experience repeated metabolic crises, which may become progressively more severe over time and result in breathing problems, seizures, brain damage, cardiac arrest or sudden death. Conservative estimates suggest that without newborn screening, at least half of children born with MCADD will have a metabolic crisis and between one in four and up to one in five will die or experience severe disability (Grosse *et al.*, 2006; Wilcken *et al.*, 2007).

The primary focus of treatment is to avoid low blood sugar. Identifying newborns affected by MCADD allows parents to manage their baby's diet and ensure a regular, adequate energy intake for their child, thereby reducing the chances of severe, life-threatening episodes of illness. Parents are taught an emergency regime to be used if the baby is unwell or not feeding. Glucose polymer feeds are given to provide energy (Dixon, 2007).

The quality of the blood spot sample, correct identification of the baby by use of the baby's NHS number and timeliness of taking and processing of the sample are vital to the blood spot programme. Thousands of babies are rescreened every year due to failure to get an adequate sample, taking the sample too early or too soon after transfusion, and delay due to the omission of vital information. For evidence-based guidelines on taking the blood spot sample, see **www.newbornbloodspot.screening.nhs.uk**. You should not undertake blood spot screening until you have received appropriate training in how to undertake the blood test as babies' feet are sensitive and may be permanently damaged from an incorrect technique. Not obtaining an appropriate blood sample may lead to an inaccurate result or a test that needs to be repeated. For further information on how to perform the blood spot screening test please visit the following website: **www.newbornbloodspot.screening.nhs.uk**

Key points
- All parents in the UK are offered screening for their baby.
- The health care practitioner should always obtain informed consent from parents prior to undertaking any neonatal screening.
- All information given to parents in relation to newborn screening should be given in a form that they are able to understand.
- The initial examination by the midwife aims to reassure parents that their baby appears normal and to detect any major physical abnormalities or problems that need immediate referral.
- The physical newborn examination is a more detailed examination of the baby, looking in particular for congenital heart defects, developmental dysplasia of the hips and congenital cataracts.
- The newborn hearing screening is undertaken to enable the detection of bilateral permanent hearing impairment.
- Newborn blood spot screening identifies babies who may have rare but serious conditions.

- The health care practitioner should only undertake screening tests that they have been fully trained to undertake.

Exercises
1. You need to obtain informed consent from parents to undertake the initial examination of the newborn. How would you obtain this – what information would you give to the parents?
2. You are working with the midwife who is about to undertake the newborn blood spot screening. The mother asks you what the test screens for. What information will you need to give her?

REFERENCES

Ainsworth, S.B., Wyllie, J.P. and Wren, C. (1999) 'Prevalence and clinical significance of cardiac murmurs in neonates'. *Archive of Disease in Childhood, Fetal Neonatal Edition.* 1999, 80: F43–45

Baston, H. and Durward, H. (2001) *Examination of the Newborn. A Practical Guide.* London: Routledge

Chan, A., McCaul, K., Cundy, P., Haan, E. and Byron-Scott, R. (1997) 'Perinatal Risk Factors for Developmental Dysplasia of the Hip'. *Archive of Disease in Childhood, Fetal Neonatal Edition,* 76: F94–100 (March)

Child Growth Foundation and Royal College of Paediatrics and Child Health. (2004) *My personal child health record.* South Shields: Harlow Printing Ltd

CNST (2004) 'Clinical Negligence Scheme for Trusts: Maternity Clinical Risk Management Standards'. NHS Litigation Authority, April 2004

Davis, A., Bamford, J. and Wilson, I. (1997) 'A critical review of the role of neonatal hearing screening in the detection of congenital hearing impairment'. *Health Technology Assessment Review* 1997, 1 (10)

Dezateux, C., Brown, J., Arthur, R., Karnon, J. and Parnaby, A. (2003) 'Performance, treatment pathways, and effects of alternative policy options for screening for developmental dysplasia of the hip in the United Kingdom'. *Arch Dis Child* 88: 753–759

DH (2001) *Good Practice in Consent: HSC2001/023*. London: Department of Health November 2001

DH (2004) Core Standards document, *National Service Framework for Children, Young People and Maternity Services*. London: Department of Health and Department for Education and Skills

DH (2007) *Collaborative Commissioning of National Screening Programmes Best Practice Guidance*. Gateway reference: 8829

Dixon, M. (2007) 'MCADD, Dietary management guidelines for dieticians'. This document is supported by the British Inherited Metabolic Disease Group. Available from **www.bimdg.org.uk** or **www.newborn bloodspot.screening.nhs.uk**

Elbourne, D., Dezateux, C., Arthur, R., Clarke, N.M.P., Gray, A., King, A., Quinn, A., Gardner, F. and Russell, G. (2002) 'Ultrasonography in the diagnosis and management of developmental dysplasia of the hip (UK Hip Trial): clinical and economic results of a multi-centre randomised controlled trial'. *The Lancet*, 360: 2009–2017

Farrell, P.M., Kosorok, M.R, Rock, M.J., Lavoxa, A., Zeng, L., Lai, H.C, Hoffman, G., Laessig, R.H., Splaingard, M.L. and the Wisconsin Cystic Fibrosis Neonatal Study Group (2001) 'Early diagnosis of cystic fibrosis through neonatal screening prevents severe malnutrition and improves long-term growth'. *Pediatrics*, 107 (1): 1–13

FASP (2007) 'Fetal Anomoly Screening Programme. What is Down's syndrome?' **http://nscfa.web.its.manchester.ac.uk/screening#fileid134** (accessed 7 February 2008)

French, L.M. and Dietz, F.R. (1999) 'Screening for developmental dysplasia of the hip'. *American Family Physician*, July 1999

Goss, P.W. (2002) 'Successful screening for neonatal hip instability in Australia'. *Journal of Paediatrics and Child Health*, 38(5): 469–474

Grosse, S. D., Khoury, M.J., Greene, C. L., Crider, K.S. and Pollitt, R.J. (2006) 'The epidemiology of medium chain acyl-CoA dehydrogenase deficiency: an update'. *Genetics in Medicine*, 8(4): 205–212

Hall, M.B. and Elliman, D. (2004) *Health for All Children* (4th Ed.). Oxford: Oxford University Press

Harcombe, J. (2007) 'Supporting midwives in screening'. *RCM Midwives*, 10 (1)

Jones, D.A. (1998) *Hip Screening in the Newborn: A practical guide.* Oxford: Butterworth Heinemann

Kanneh, A. and Davies, F. (2000) 'Physical characteristics and physiological features of a full term neonate: Theory practice integration part 1'. *Journal of Advanced Neonatal Nursing*, 6 (1): 4–13

Kelsberg, G., Bishop, R. and Morton, J. (2006). 'When should a child with an undescended testis be referred to an urologist?' *Journal of Family Practice*, 55(4): 336–337 **www.jfponline.com/Pages.asp?AID= 4013&UID**

Knowles, R., Griebsch, I., Dezateux, C., Brown, J., Bull, C. and Wren, C. (2005) 'Newborn screening for congenital heart defects; a systematic review and cost effectiveness analysis'. *Health Technology Assessment* 2005

NDCS (2005) 'Understanding deafness. An introductory guide to different types of deafness; hearing tests; communication and language'. National Deaf Children's Society, February 2005

NHS QIS (2004) 'Routine examination of the newborn. Best practice statement'. NHS Quality Improvement Scotland 2004

NHS Sickle and Thalassaemia screening programme (2006) *Standards for the Linked Antenatal and Newborn Screening Programme.* Available from **http://sct.screening.nhs.uk/publications.htm**

NICE (2003) *Antenatal care: Routine care for the healthy pregnant woman.* Clinical guideline 6. London: NICE

NICE (2006) *Postnatal care: Routine postnatal care of women and their babies.* Clinical guideline 37. London: NICE

NICE (2007) *Intrapartum care: Care of healthy women and their babies during childbirth.* Clinical guideline 5. London: NICE

NSC (2003) *Criteria for appraising the viability, effectiveness and appropriateness of a screening programme.* National Screening Committee. March 2003

NSC (2004) *Child Health Sub-group Report Dysplasia of the Hip.* September 2004.

NSC (2005) 'Child Health Sub-group Committee on Congenital Cataract'

NSC (2006a) 'National Screening Committee policy – Congenital Cataract Screening'. July 2006. **www.library.nhs.uk/screening/ViewResource.aspx?resID=57177&tab ID=288&catID=2012** (accessed 6 February 2008)

NSC (2006b) *Cryptochordism screening.* National Screening Committee policy–July 2006 **www.library.nhs.uk/screening/ViewResource.aspx?res ID=57178&tabID=288&catID=2015**

Park, M. K. (2002) *Pediatric cardiology for practitioners* (4th Ed.). St Louis: Mosby

Pollitt, R.J., Green, A., McCabe, A. *et al.* (1997) 'Neonatal screening for inborn errors of metabolism: cost, yield and outcome'. *Health Technology Assessment*, 1: 1–203

Raffle, A. and Gray, M. (2007) *Screening. Evidence and Practice.* Oxford: Oxford University Press

Rahi, J.S. and Dezateux, C. (1999). 'National Cross Sectional Study of Detection of Congenital and Infantile Cataract in the United Kingdom: Role of Childhood Screening and Surveillance. The British Congenital Cataract Interest Group'. *British Medical Journal*, 318 (7180): 362–365

RCOG (2000) 'Ultrasound Screening' supplement to *Ultrasound Screening for Fetal Abnormalities* **www.rcog.org.uk/index.asp?PageID= 1185#app1** (accessed 3 February 2008)

Robins, J. (2001) 'Congenital cataract: The role of the neonatal nurse practitioner in screening and provision of psychological support'. *Journal of Neonatal Nursing,* 7(3): 91–94

Rock, M.J. (2007) 'Newborn screening for cystic fibrosis'. *Clinics in Chest Medicine,*28(2): 297–305

Seymour, C.A., Thomason, M.J., Chalmers, R.A., Addison, G.M., Bain, M.D., Cockburn, F. *et al.* (1997) 'Newborn screening for inborn errors of metabolism: a systematic review'. *Health Technology Assessment* 1997, 1(11).

Stewart, R., Hargreaves, K. and Oliver, S. (2004) 'Telling parents about the heel-prick test: consultation results and resource development', 1–49. London: UK Newborn Screening Programme Centre.

Tappero, E.P. and Honeyfield, M.E. (2003) *Physical assessment of the newborn* (3rd Ed.). Santa Rosa, CA: NICU INK

Townsend, J., Wolke, D., Hayes, J., Dave, S., Rogers, C., Bloomfield, L., Quist-Therson, E., Tomlin, M. and Messer, D. (2004) EMREN – *Evaluation of midwives' role extension in the routine examination of the newborn*. Health Technology Assessment NHS R&D HTA Programme

UKNSPC (2005) *Health Professional Handbook: Informed choice and communicating with parents*. UK Newborn Screening Programme Centre, April 2005

UKNSPC (2005) 'Newborn blood spot screening in the UK', *Health professional handbook*. UK Newborn Screening Programme Centre, April 2005

Wilcken, B., Haas, M., Joy, P., Wiley, V., Chaplin, M., Black, C. *et al.* (2007) 'Outcome of neonatal screening for medium-chain acyl-CoA dehydrogenase deficiency in Australia: a cohort study'. The *Lancet* 369(9555): 37–42

Witt, C. (2003) 'Detecting Developmental Dysplasia of the Hip'. *Advances in Neonatal Care*, 3 (2): 65–75

Useful Websites

www.screening.nhs.uk/cpd/index.htm

Chapter 5

Principles of Feeding
Karen Hill

Chapter aims

To explore the current knowledge and recommendations in relation to feeding practices that maximise health benefits to neonates.

Learning outcomes

By the end of this chapter you will be able to:

- demonstrate knowledge of the basic anatomy and physiology of the breast;
- discuss current findings, the physiology of lactation and factors that promote breastfeeding;
- describe the WHO/UNICEF baby-friendly recommendations and initiatives to promote successful breastfeeding;
- demonstrate an understanding of feeding methods for both the 'normal' neonate and those neonates with special requirements;
- discuss the role of voluntary organisations, peer support and breastfeeding cafes.

Mapping to standards of proficiency
Standards of Proficiency for Pre-registration Midwifery Education (SPME)
Determine and provide programmes of care and support of women which includes consideration for – plans for feeding their babies.

Standards of Proficiency for Pre-registration Nursing Education
Provide relevant and current health information to patients, clients and groups in a form which facilitates their understanding and acknowledges choice/individual preference.

INTRODUCTION

Infant feeding has always been a contentious and sometimes quite thorny issue. The benefits of breastfeeding are highlighted to health professionals and the slogan 'breast is best' is familiar to us. The concept of human milk for human babies seems rational and breastfeeding is the physiological way to feed the young infant (Lawson, 2007). No other mammal is even capable of feeding its young with artificial milk. However, as health professionals we must ensure that information is provided and that women are able to make an informed choice. That choice, once made, should be respected and the woman should have the support of the professional in her decision.

There will also be times when other issues come into play that may affect the method by which a baby is fed and these must be understood with a view to supporting the mother and providing for the baby in the most appropriate way for its needs.

This chapter will explore feeding methods for both the 'normal' (full term, uncomplicated) baby and those babies that have special requirements. This will include breastfeeding, artificial feeding, the need and use of naso-gastric tube feeding and some problems that can occur in the baby that may affect baby's ability to feed or be fed. To understand breastfeeding, it is important to gain knowledge of the anatomy and physiology of the breast and the physiology of lactation and this will also be covered within this chapter.

ANATOMY AND PHYSIOLOGY OF THE BREAST

The usual positioning of the female breast is on each side of the chest between the second and sixth rib space. The breasts lie over the pectoralis major muscle and are held in place by suspensory ligaments.

The gross anatomy of the breast features three main areas that act as points of reference for the underlying structures and also have an important part to play in the 'art' of breastfeeding, which will be discussed later in this chapter.

- The axillary tail is the edge of the breast tissue that extends up to the axilla (under the arm).
- The areola is the pigmented circular area in the middle of the breast. Colours of this vary depending on the colour of the skin.
- The nipple is a protrusion in the centre of the areola, made up of highly sensitive pigmented erectile tissue. It contains a multitude of small openings, where the lactiferous ducts come to the surface. These are covered by epithelium.

Under the surface of the skin, the breast is mostly made up of glandular and fatty tissue. Each breast is divided into lobes. Each lobe is a self-contained unit with the structures required for milk production during and after pregnancy.

- Alveoli – each of these is lined with milk-secreting cells (acini) which are able to create milk from the factors taken from the maternal blood supply to the breast.
- Lactiferous tubules – these are small 'pipes' which connect the alveoli.
- Lactiferous duct – this is a central, larger 'pipe' that the tubules empty into. There is also a continuation of the lactiferous duct after the ampulla that extends to the opening on the nipple.
- Ampulla – a widened 'pooling' area in the lactiferous duct where milk is stored until its release.

Breast development begins for both males and females in uterine life at around the fourth week and continues throughout the life of the fetus. At birth the breast tissue can sometimes be enlarged due to the effects of the mother's hormones. This can happen in both male and female babies and parents should be reassured that it is normal and will only last a few days. This is the last breast tissue activity until puberty (Verrals, 1997).

At puberty, due to the rise in hormone levels, the breast tissue of the female develops further. At first this is due to rising oestrogen levels and then to rising progesterone levels, leading to growth of the lactiferous ducts, pronouncement of the nipple and areola and then to multiplying growth of the alveoli. The overall amounts of fat and fibrous tissue are also increased, and this is what leads in the most part to the increase in breast size. At points through their menstrual cycle, women of childbearing age often experience breast changes that are similar in part to those experienced during pregnancy. These are caused by changes in hormone secretion (progesterone) and subside again once menstruation has occurred.

In pregnancy, breast changes are often one of the first signs that the body is changing. Hormonal changes (increases in oestrogens) stimulate further development of the nipple, areola, lactiferous tubules and ducts. Further increases in the number of alveoli occur, to ready themselves for milk production; they then enlarge and again increase in number (progesterone from the corpus luteum at first and then from the developing placenta). After 16 weeks' gestation, true colostrum is often seen (yellow in colour and creamy in consistency) but this may have been preceded a few weeks earlier by a clear watery fluid as the secreting structures and lactiferous tubules and ducts prepare for the flow of milk once the baby is born (Verrals, 1997)

Once breastfeeding has been commenced and the milk supply is being maintained, the breasts can be thought of as fully functioning organs as it is at this time only that they are being utilised to their full potential and undertaking the role for which they have prepared.

After the birth of a baby, lactation will occur in all but a very small percentage of women, as it is a normal physiological phenomenon instigated once the baby is expelled. For the mother to breastfeed successfully, lactation must be maintained, and the mechanisms important for this can be affected by outside influences as diverse as maternal illness or societal perceptions. These factors will be discussed later in the chapter.

Physiology of lactation

The production of milk within the breast and the passage of that milk through the breast to the baby are governed by hormonal control. The hormone essential for the production of milk is prolactin (secreted by the anterior pituitary gland in the brain). The level of this rises throughout pregnancy but other pregnancy hormones (those from the placenta) suppress its action while the pregnancy is still ongoing. Once the pregnancy is over and the baby, placenta and membranes have been delivered, the pregnancy hormones gradually decrease and the levels of prolactin begin to be effective in the production of milk as its levels and actions are less and less suppressed. The blood supply through the breast increases and the constituents that are essential for milk production are extracted from the maternal blood. The acini cells are distended by protein molecules and fatty globules and the resulting product is squeezed out into the lactiferous tubules. All is now ready for the passage of milk for the baby.

Figure 5.1 below shows a simplified drawing of the breast during lactation. You can see that the key structures have become enlarged (distended) to allow for the production of milk. Figure 5.2 shows an enlargement of the alveoli and their place within the breast lobe (C).

From the figures below it is easy to see how the passage of milk may be facilitated by the physical structures of the breast.

The hormonal influences are the stimulation for that process to take place for the most part although, as mentioned previously, the acini cells are distended with their protein/fatty globule production and some of the globules are forced out into the lactiferous tubules through 'overcrowding' in the acini cell.

The hormone responsible for the passage of milk is oxytocin (secreted by the posterior pituitary gland in the brain). This hormone is stimulated by the baby's sucking at the breast which causes an unconditioned reflex within the pituitary gland and the oxytocin is released. The oxytocin

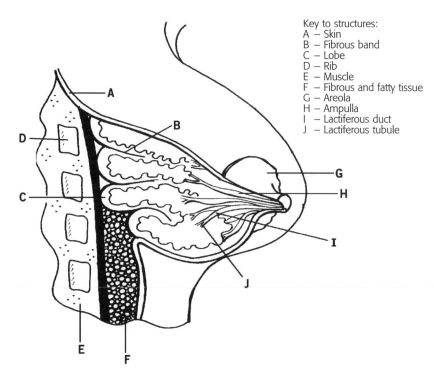

Key to structures:
A – Skin
B – Fibrous band
C – Lobe
D – Rib
E – Muscle
F – Fibrous and fatty tissue
G – Areola
H – Ampulla
I – Lactiferous duct
J – Lactiferous tubule

Figure 5.1 The anatomy of the breast

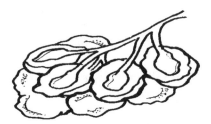

Figure 5.2 The alveoli

works directly on the alveolus as each one is surrounded by a contractile cell network that responds to it and squeezes the milk out into the lactiferous tubules. It then flows to the ampulla and then to the baby via the nipple end of the lactiferous duct. This mechanism is often referred to as the 'let-down' reflex.

Research undertaken by Ramsay *et al.* (2005) using ultrasound imaging has reported changes to the breast anatomy during lactation that suggest that the anatomy of the breast in lactating women is different from that which has been previously understood and described. The significant changes are:

- lactiferous ducts branch closer to the nipple;
- lactiferous sinuses (ampulla) do not exist as previously thought;
- glandular tissue is found closer to the nipple;
- there is minimal subcutaneous fat at the base of the nipple.

It should be mentioned here that oxytocin is also the hormone responsible for uterine contraction and so, with its release while feeding, mothers will often experience some abdominal discomfort as the uterus contracts back to its pre-pregnant state (these are often referred to as 'after pains').

Maintenance of lactation relies on supply and demand. The baby feeding at the breast will stimulate ongoing production of milk and the more that he or she is put to the breast, the more milk will be produced. In this way, it is easy to see that a mother breastfeeding twins will be able to produce enough to satisfy both babies.

The way that the baby attaches to the breast and therefore sucks is important for the maintenance of lactation. The baby should envelop most of the areola with its mouth and, in doing this, the gums will apply pressure within the breast and so will force the milk out to the surface of the breast. Sucking just at the nipple will not result in the baby's stimulating the breast to produce an adequate supply of milk and, in most cases, will lead to discomfort and damage to the nipple if prolonged. If a mother reports discomfort throughout the feed, or finds it 'too painful' to breastfeed, this will most likely be due to poor attachment, and she should be offered help and support to overcome this.

It is also important that the baby is fed from one breast for one feed in its entirety. Previously it was thought that this was so that the baby gets both the fore and the richer hind milk with each feed. However, Ramsay's research (2005) suggests that there is no 'fore' or 'hind' milk but that the constituents of the milk change to suit the needs of the baby. This is consistent with other findings regarding the constituents of breast milk, as well as with the work undertaken by some artificial food manufacturers. If the baby is still hungry after one breast but has unattached itself, it is good practice to advise that the baby be put to the other breast for the remainder of the feed (NICE, 2006) but that they start with the second breast for the next complete feed. For example:

- feed one: right breast offered for feed – baby removes itself from the breast but still appears interested in feeding – left breast offered – baby feeds and falls asleep;
- feed two: left breast offered for feed.

CURRENT GUIDANCE ON BREASTFEEDING

In 1992 UNICEF and the World Health Organization (WHO) launched the Baby Friendly Initiative (BFI) to encourage maternity hospitals to implement the 'Ten steps to successful breastfeeding' and, in 1994, it was launched in the UK. These ten steps and the later introduced 'Seven Point Plan for the Protection, Promotion and Support of Breastfeeding in Community Healthcare Settings' (UNICEF/WHO, 1998) are still seen by many as the gold standard for breastfeeding support. The aim is to ensure that pregnant and breastfeeding women have access to a high standard of care by supporting health care facilities seeking to implement best practice within their units. It also offers an assessment and accreditation process to recognise those who achieve the standards.

The steps are focused on the health care providers (acute hospitals, community care settings) and the practitioners who work within them to enable them to offer the necessary best practice to this client group. They have formed the basis of many maternity units' approach to the care and support of breastfeeding since their launch, even in units that have not achieved full accreditation, and have also informed subsequent nationally recognised guidance and standards.

In 2006 the National Institute for Health and Clinical Excellence (NICE) issued guidance surrounding routine postnatal care for women and their babies. Included within this guidance is information regarding infant feeding and recommendations for best practice. Much of this guidance can be seen to mirror the best practice standards set out in the earlier UNICEF standards. Maternity units should also have their own local policies or guidelines to lead health care practitioners to appropriate practice within their own units and enable them to highlight specific areas for practice within that locality. This may be taking into account a particular cultural aspect, a particular population of women or just information regarding the demographics of the area. Local guidelines should be informed from recognised sources such as the NICE guidelines and that of the UNICEF Baby Friendly Initiative to ensure that best practice is recommended. Any health care practitioners commencing work in a particular area should ensure that they are familiar with local as well as national guidance.

Information box 1

The NICE guidance outlines six headings under the 'Infant feeding' section that proposes recommendations for the health care professional working with the breastfeeding mother. These are:

- a supportive environment for breastfeeding;
- starting successful breastfeeding;
- continuing successful breastfeeding;
- assessing successful breastfeeding;
- expression and storage of breast milk;
- preventing, identifying and treating breastfeeding concerns.

(NICE, 2006 1.3, pp. 20–26)

Much of the guidance offered under these headings consists of mechanisms that are routinely offered in most maternity units and community settings, but setting them out in this format allows units to ensure that what they are offering remains best practice and has not become ritual rather than evidence-based. It is not very often that, when asked why something is done a particular way, the answer 'because we have always done it that way' is appropriate. In the busy acute settings where most women have their babies, time is the most precious commodity. Whether it is the time that health care practitioners have to care for the women and their babies, time that the family have together without interruptions, time that the woman spends breastfeeding, or just time for the mother to spend gazing at her wonderful new baby, it is a feature of care that can quite easily be eroded. This may be the reason that many of the points issued in the NICE guidelines are time related and highlight the importance of this aspect of care and the need to ensure that all families have the requisite time for each and every activity related to breastfeeding that is practicable. The issue of initial contact between mother and baby and timing of the first feed has raised much discussion and much is written about this area of care. UNICEF (1992) state in Point Four of their ten steps '…help mothers to initiate breastfeeding soon after birth'. NICE (2006, p. 21) goes a step further by stating that 'initiation of breastfeeding should be encouraged [as] soon after the birth, ideally within one hour' and that, along with this, mothers should be encouraged to have skin-to-skin contact with their babies as soon as possible after the birth. This is a view that is shared by Colson (2007) who states, in her work on biological nurturing, that encouraging mother–baby separation has a detrimental effect on both milk production and potentially on the metabolic adaptation of the baby. She goes further than the NICE guidance in recommending that mothers are informed of the benefits of 'baby holding' over and above the first hour, to ensure that the breast is accessible for frequent small feeds, even when the baby is sleeping.

Providing a supportive environment for breastfeeding to start and continue successfully should be at the forefront of care planning for the postnatal woman and her family within any setting and is supported by both the UNICEF standards and by the NICE guidance.

FACTORS INFLUENCING BREASTFEEDING

Despite being a normal physiological phenomenon, there are many factors that can influence successful breastfeeding. These can range from intrinsic factors relating to the mother's body or physical condition, to societal or cultural factors. The promotion of breastfeeding depends on the health care practitioner having an understanding of these factors and the effect that they can have on the mother and her baby.

The following factors are not an exhaustive list. There may be particular factors that promote breastfeeding for just one woman and, as with other areas of care, there should be an individualised approach, taking the unique experience of a particular family into account.

Information box 2

Factors known to promote breastfeeding
- Privacy – irrespective of whether in hospital or at home. The woman should feel secure in her environment.
- Information – from health care practitioners, family, peers, society.
- Comfort – including good patterns of rest for the mother as well as the position in which to feed.
- Knowledge – of why 'breast is best' and the constituents contained in breast milk and their function.
- Convenience – time and money can be saved by not having to buy artificial formula or get up to make a feed.
- Bonding – unique time spent with her baby and a chance to 'get to know' them.
- Health benefits – return of pre-pregnant body image sooner. Reduced risk of breast and ovarian cancer (Medforth *et al.*, 2006).
- Contraception – high levels of the hormone prolactin suppress ovulation in a mother who is fully breastfeeding.
- Support – from partners, family and friends as well as peer groups. Introduction of 'baby cafes' and peer support groups for target groups such as, for example, teenage mothers/socially excluded should not be underestimated (Medforth *et al.*, 2006).

Information box 3

Factors known to inhibit breastfeeding.

- Pain – known to inhibit the release of oxytocin, thus the 'let-down reflex' is inhibited.
- Inconsistent advice – many mothers site this reason for difficulty in establishing breastfeeding (Medforth *et al.*, 2006).
- Reduced haemoglobin levels – due to poor diet, non-compliance with iron supplementation, large blood loss at delivery.
- Body image – the breasts seen as a sex symbol rather than as a feeding organ (Verrals, 1997).
- Society views – mothers may have been asked not to feed in public places.
- Lack of knowledge – 34 per cent of women believe modern formula milks are very similar to breast milk (DH, 2004a).
- Health myths – 20 per cent of 16–24-year-old women believe that breastfeeding will ruin the shape of their breasts/bodies (DH, 2004a).
- Peer pressure – mothers are surrounded by others who are not breast-feeding and who are often perpetuating myths.
- Pacifiers (dummies) – no strong evidence exists regarding the effects of these on the initiation of breastfeeding but there is concern by UNICEF BFI (1992) that there is a link and this is a view shared by many health care practitioners.

INSTANCES WHERE BREASTFEEDING MAY BE CONTRAINDICATED

Breastfeeding is the best way for a mother to feed her new baby but, as stated in the introduction to this chapter, there are some times when this is either not possible or the woman has chosen not to breastfeed. While virtually all women can breastfeed (DH, 2004a), there are some instances in which breastfeeding becomes either more complicated or is contra-indicated. The next few paragraphs highlight some of these instances, and these issues, along with the individual woman's choice, may influence the way in which her baby is fed.

Maternal causes

Drugs

Some drugs – either prescription or illicit drugs – affect breastfeeding. Many drugs pass into the breast milk and therefore on to the baby, and the health care practitioner should be aware of those that may cause a problem. Many drugs are perfectly safe to take both in pregnancy and while breastfeeding, and GPs will often attempt to prescribe less harmful drugs if they are necessary throughout pregnancy and breastfeeding, and also consider whether the benefits of taking them outweigh the risks. This may be particularly relevant in drugs such as some antidepressants (British National Formulary (BNF), 2007) or cancer-treating drugs that are highly toxic (Medforth *et al.*, 2006) and the midwife should be aware of the effects that any drugs may have. Health care professionals need to know that there are other sources of information and who they can ask for advice about drugs and breastfeeding. This may be specialist midwives whose remit is to work with pregnant women who are using illicit drugs, or members of the pharmacy staff who provide a valuable source of information.

Breast surgery

Breast surgery – whether for medical or cosmetic reasons – is not always a contraindication to breastfeeding but knowledge of the surgical technique would be necessary and advice should be sought from the surgeon.

HIV infection

In the UK and other developed countries current advice is that HIV-positive mothers should not breastfeed (to decrease the potential risk of vertical transmission – mother to baby) but should use an appropriate infant formula from birth (DH, 2004b). In developing countries where there is a risk of unsafe formula preparation practices, due to the inability to ensure clean water supplies, breastfeeding is still advocated and a study by Coovadia *et al.* (2007) highlighted that the transmission rate from mother to baby in exclusively breastfed babies where the mother was known to be HIV positive was approximately four per cent only and their study suggested that this should lead to revision of the guidelines on this as published by UNICEF and WHO. It should also be considered that there may be times within our own society when clean water may be an issue. This could be with travelling families where there is no running water available or, potentially, in families that rely on well water rather than a mains supply. The Environment Agency issues guidance on this each year so that health care professionals are aware of the issues involved.

Neonatal causes

- **Prematurity** – if a baby is premature, ill or weak, it is sometimes not possible for them to feed from the breast, and other methods may have to be adopted (naso-gastric feeding or cup feeding). The baby can be fed expressed breast milk in this way.

- **Facial anomalies** – babies with small chins (micrognathia) or tongue-tie (ankyloglossia) may experience difficulty feeding effectively (DH, 2006).
- **Hypoglycaemia** – a significant drop in the baby's blood sugar can affect its ability to wake for effective feeding. This may be due to the effects of a difficult delivery (babies that require resuscitation will have used a far greater amount of their glucose stores – Resuscitation Council UK, 2006) or because the baby has a diabetic mother (see Chapter 8).

ARTIFICIAL FEEDING

All pregnant women should be informed of the benefits of breastfeeding but, if the woman chooses to bottle feed her baby, guidance should be given to ensure that she does so safely (DH, 2006; Medforth *et al.*, 2006).

The main difference between breast milk and formula milk is the constituents contained within them. Breast milk is a dynamic fluid, the composition of which changes during the course of lactation, and it is biologically complex – with 300 components within its constitution (Lawson, 2007). It would be impossible for manufacturers of formula milk to reproduce this but the constituents of modern formula have changed over the years to attempt to get close to those in breast milk. They can never hope to replicate many of the ingredients such as antibodies, hormones and live cells, but the aim is to try to support the growth and development of the baby and to try and mimic physiological responses in the baby that are similar to those apparent in breastfed babies.

There are many differences between breast and formula milk but the most commonly quoted difference is the protein content within the two. The protein content of formula milk has historically been more similar to that of cow's milk, which contains a higher proportion of casein (the curds) than the whey content, and so is more difficult for the new baby to break down and digest. Breast milk is higher in whey content and so is more easily assimilated by the digestive system. Modern formulas are now able to match the whey to casein proportions of mature breast milk (60:40) but are still unable to match the types of proteins into which they are further broken down.

Alpha-lactalbumin (alpha-protein), which is the predominant whey protein in breast milk, plays an important part in babies' nutrition, growth and development and is a source of essential amino acids. This is the only whey protein in breast milk. Beta-lactoglobulin (beta-protein) is the predominant whey protein in cow's milk and is currently the predominant whey protein in formula milk. It does not occur in breast milk. It is this constituent that formula feed manufacturers are trying to decrease in an attempt to mimic breast milk more closely (SMA, 2007).

The advertising of artificial formula is closely monitored to ensure that formula is not advocated over breast milk as being best for the baby. Stricter controls on the labelling of packaging were introduced in 2008 to ensure that parents are able to clearly identify the difference between first milk and follow-on milk (DH, 2008).

Women who are artificially feeding need to be made aware of the current recommendations for preparing formula feeds as these have changed. Many women rely on their families for support when they have a new baby and the midwife should be aware that there is a potential for misinformation through this route as outdated practices may be passed on as the most appropriate way to do things. All dry powdered formula feeds marketed in the UK are prepared in the same way, using 30 ml of cooled boiled tap water with one level scoop of milk powder added. The water should be cooled for 30 minutes following boiling. Baby milk powder is not sterile and as it is a food source it is an excellent medium for bacteria and microbes to grow and multiply (Food Standards Agency, 2007), so it is essential that good hygiene practices are adhered to and that the mother is aware of these (Lawson, 2007). The current recommendations are that only one feed is prepared at a time and, where it is not practical to prepare a feed on demand, a feed can be prepared and stored in the main body of a fridge, following quick cooling, and then transported in a cool bag to be used within four hours of preparation (Food Standards Agency, 2006). The Department of Health (2006) recognises that it is essential for mothers who choose to bottle feed their babies to be given appropriate advice and support.

BABIES WITH SPECIAL FEEDING REQUIREMENTS

Naso-gastric (NG) feeding

For some babies there may be problems with feeding from the breast (suck feeding) due to prematurity or illness. In these instances they may need to have their food delivered direct to their stomach and this is done via a naso-gastric (NG) tube. If mothers are planning to breastfeed they should be supported in expressing breast milk and this may be given via the tube. Babies who require tube feeding are those who are unable to maintain full nutrition by breast or bottle alone. In premature babies this may be due to their neurological immaturity affecting their ability to suck.

When inserting a naso-gastric tube into the baby's stomach, it is important that the tube is first measured against the size of the baby so that it is inserted at the correct length. It should be measured from the tip of the xiphisternum to the tragus of the ear and across to the nostrils (the tragus being the fleshy part at the front of the ear). You should not undertake the passing of a nao-gastric tube until you have been fully trained and assessed.

The baby should be relaxed and warm prior to the procedure. It should take at least 15 seconds to pass the tube into the stomach in order to prevent vagal stimulation and a possible bradycardia. Once the tube is inserted, gastric acidity should be checked to ensure that the tube is in the stomach and has not been inadvertently passed into the lung via the left main brochus. This is done by putting a small amount of aspirate onto an appropriate pH indicator paper. A result of 5.5 or less should indicate correct placement; 6–6.5 could indicate intestinal pH and indicate that the tube is too long; and a pH of 7 could indicate a lung pH and feed should not be given down the tube in this instance. (National patient Safety Agency (2005) Patient Safety Alert NPSA/2005/9 **www.npsa.nhs. ukadvice**).

Once the NG tube is confirmed in the correct position, feeding can commence and this should be done via an oral syringe attached to the end of the feeding tube. The feed should be allowed to flow by gravity down the tube and should not be pushed down with the aid of the plunger (although this may be needed to start the flow). It is recognised that the longer babies are without suck feeding, the poorer their feeding may be at a later date (Bagnall, 2005).

It should be noted here that, due to a National Patient Safety Agency (NPSA) directive that came into force in March 2008, only syringes designated for the giving of oral and enteral feeding should be used for the administration of NG feeds.

Cup feeding

In a baby who is temporarily unable to feed at the breast, cup feeding offers an alternative that does not lead to the introduction of an artificial teat. It sometimes works as a useful follow-on from a naso-gastric tube (particularly one that has been in place for some time) to breastfeeding as it encourages the suck/swallow/breathing co-ordination (Medforth et al., 2006). It is important that mothers are taught the correct technique: the baby should 'lap' at the cup rather than the milk be poured into its mouth. Mothers should also be warned that a higher than usual spillage rate should be expected, even when proficiently cup feeding, and reminded that this should be taken into account when calculating the amount of milk that the baby has had.

FEEDING SUPPORT ORGANISATIONS AND GROUPS

There are many support organisations nationally and locally. These range from those set up as a resource for mothers and health care practitioners to gain access to the most up-to-date information, to independent peer support groups set up in local areas to offer support through access to others in the same situation.

The National Childbirth Trust (NCT) is a national organisation that has many local groups and trains its own breastfeeding counsellors who act as a point of contact for any specific feeding problems. These are all mothers who have breastfed themselves and can therefore share their knowledge and experience with new mothers who may be experiencing difficulties. The NCT also provide a wealth of information leaflets for mothers and fathers on issues surrounding feeding (**www.nct.org.uk**).

In many local areas, groups of mothers have set up support groups to help each other with problems and also to develop a social network of like-minded people. Increasingly, these are taking the form of 'baby cafes' that are places where mothers can take their babies, meet friends and know that they can feed their babies while enjoying the social side of the cafe culture too. Some of these baby cafes are facilitated by local county councils or are run through community midwifery teams, and others are independently run by local mothers.

In some areas there are groups that have been set up to target specific categories of mothers who may ordinarily not access support of this nature or who are within a marginalised population. They may be teenage mothers, mothers from a particular ethnic background, or mothers who speak only a particular non-English language. Sure Start schemes have provided much-needed support in some of these areas.

Many community midwifery teams also run breastfeeding workshops in the antenatal period for women to attend before their babies arrive. All women are encouraged to attend these, even if they are undecided on their chosen method of feeding, as they are a good way of accessing support through a peer group, and also provide access to health care practitioners with a special interest in the subject.

Publications are also available to offer support and some further points of contact available are:

- La Leche League – **www.laleche.org.uk**
- Breastfeeding Network – **www.breastfeedingnetwork.org.uk**
- UNICEF Baby Friendly Initiative – **www.babyfriendly.org.uk**

This is not an exhaustive list and there are many other organisations, including local county council information services, that offer support and information about what is available for mothers in any particular locality.

SUMMARY

This chapter has looked in some detail at the issues surrounding feeding a newborn baby. It has provided the anatomy and physiology necessary to begin to understand the changes within the body in response to pregnancy and through which the body begins the lactation process. The information given has attempted to be unbiased and, while recognising the importance of breastfeeding, has attempted to provide the reader with sufficient access to information to enable them to support a woman through making feeding choices and encountering any difficulties, and to recognise the unique and privileged position in which they, as a health care practitioner, find themselves.

Key points
- Accurate information should be given to women about infant feeding, and a woman's choice regarding feeding her baby should be respected and supported.
- Breastfeeding ensures that the baby receives the milk that is specially produced for that purpose.
- Mothers who choose to artificially feed should be in possession of all of the facts regarding formula milk and its constituents.
- The effects of infant feeding are very much on the agenda for national/governmental bodies, and health professionals need to stay up to date with the current findings and recommendations.
- Mothers of babies with more complex feeding needs should be given the necessary support and expertise to enable them still to feel that they are able to provide for their infant.
- Support groups are available for mothers to access and peer group support appears to offer them invaluable assistance.

Exercises

1. You are the health professional allocated to caring for a mother who is unsure of how best to feed her baby and she asks you for advice. What information would you give her?

2. You visit a mother and baby at home and find that all the artificial feeds for the next two days are prepared and in the door of the fridge. How would you tackle this subject with the mother?
3. A new mother feels that she is not coping very well with feeding and is worried about what will happen when she goes home. What would your advice to her be?
4. You overhear a colleague giving outdated advice to a new mother on the postnatal ward. What would you do? You may like to consider how you would deal with a) your colleague and b) the mother that received the advice.

REFERENCES

Bagnall, A. (2005) 'Feeding Problems', in Jones, E. and King, C. *Feeding and Nutrition in the preterm infant.* London: Elsevier

British National Formulary (2007) *British National Formulary* (BNF). London: BNF Publishing Group Ltd

Colson, S. (2007) 'The physiology of lactation revisited'. *The Practising Midwife*, 10 (10): 14–19

Coovadia, H.M., Rollins, N.C., Bland, R. M., Little, K., Coutsoudis, A., Bennish, M.L. and Newell, M. (2007) 'Mother-to-child transmission of HIV-1 infection during exclusive breastfeeding in the first six months of life: an intervention cohort study'. The *Lancet*, 369: 1107–1116

Department of Health (2004a) 'Myths stop women giving babies best start in life'. *Press Release.* **www.dh.gov.uk**

Department of Health (2004b) HIV and Infant feeding. Guidance from the Chief Medical Officers' Expert Advisory Group on AIDS. London: Department of Health

Department of Health (2006) *Bottle feeding.* **www.dh.gov.uk/publications**

Department of Health (2008) 'Update on infant formula legislation'. *Maternal and Infant Nutrition.* **www.dh.gov.uk**

Food Standards (2006) *Guidance for health professionals on safe preparation, storage and handling of powdered infant formula.* **www.food.gov.uk**

Food Standards (2007) *Guidelines for making up special feeds for infants and children in hospital.* Produced by the Special Feed working group of the Paediatric Group of the British Diatetic Association. London: HM Government

Lawson, M. (2007) 'Contemporary aspects of infant feeding'. *Paediatric Nursing,* 19 (2): 39–45.

Medforth, J., Battersby, S., Evans, M., Marsh, B. and Walker, A. (2006) *Oxford Handbook of Midwifery.* Oxford: Oxford University Press

National Institute for Health and Clinical Excellence (NICE) (2006) *Routine postnatal care of women and their babies.* Clinical guideline 37. London: NICE

Ramsay, D.T., Kent, J.C., Hartmann, R.A. and Hartmann, P.E. (2005) 'Anatomy of the Human Lactating Breast redefined with ultrasound imaging'. *Journal of Anatomy,* 206: 525–534

Resuscitation Council UK (2006) *Newborn Life Support Resuscitation at Birth* (2nd Ed.). Resuscitation Council (UK)

SMA Healthcare Professionals (2007) *Alpha-lactalbumin. The most fundamental change to protein in infant formula for over three decades.* Berkshire: SMA Nutrition

UNICEF and World Health Organization (WHO) (1992) *Ten Steps to Successful Breastfeeeeding.* **www.babyfriendly.org.uk**

UNICEF and World Health Organization (WHO) (1998) *Seven Point Plan for the Protection, Promotion and Support of Breastfeeding in the Community Healthcare Setting.* **www.babyfriendly.org.uk**

Verrals, S. (1997) *Anatomy and Physiology Applied to Obstetrics* (3rd Ed.). New York: Churchill Livingstone

ACKNOWLEDGEMENTS

Many thanks to Lance Alexander for the illustrations.

Chapter 6

Assessment of Ongoing Neonatal Well-being and Advice for Parents
Amanda Williamson and Kenda Crozier

Chapter aims

To introduce you to the knowledge required to assess neonatal well-being.

Learning outcomes
By the end of this chapter you will be able to:

- discuss 'normal' behavioural and physiological parameters in babies;
- describe the health practitioner's role in the assessment and care of a baby's well-being;
- demonstrate an understanding of common minor disorders;
- discuss the advice given to help reduce the risk of sudden infant death;
- discuss the importance of early immunisation for Hepatitis B and TB.

Mapping to standards of proficiency
Standards of Proficiency for Pre-registration Midwifery Education (SPME)
Determine and provide programmes of care and support of women which includes consideration for – needs for postnatal support, preparation for parenthood needs.
Care for and monitor women during the puerperium, offering the necessary evidence-based advice and support regarding the baby and self-care. This will include:

- providing advice and support on feeding babies and teaching women about the importance of nutrition in child development;
- providing advice and support on hygiene, safety, protection, security and child development;
- enabling women to address issues about their own, their babies' and their families' health and social well-being.

Standards of Proficiency for Pre-registration Nursing education
Provide relevant and current health information to patients, clients and groups in a form which facilitates their understanding and acknowledges choice/individual preference.
Contribute to the application of a range of interventions which support and optimise the health and well-being of patients and clients.

INTRODUCTION

The National Institute for Health and Clinical Excellence Postnatal Care Guidelines say that at all postnatal visits parents should be offered advice and relevant information to enable them to assess the baby's general condition; to be able to identify signs and symptoms of common health problems seen in babies; and to know how and when to contact a health care professional or access emergency care for their baby if required (NICE, 2006). The Midwives Rules and Standards (NMC, 2004) highlight that a midwife is responsible for the woman and her baby during the postnatal period. The ongoing assessment of the baby's well-being may become the responsibility of the midwife or nurse. It is important that as you go through your training you learn to 'baby watch'. Ensuring that you spend time actually looking at normal babies and their behaviour will help you to identify when a baby may need extra care or is ill.

Parents may be confused by the array of conflicting advice about normal behaviour patterns that is available through the media from a range of 'baby experts'. Therefore it is important that health professionals are able to give clear advice and answer questions. This chapter will enable you to answer some questions and decide when to refer parents to others for advice or help.

INITIAL ASSESSMENT

The first stage of assessment of well-being may be undertaken by talking to the mother and her partner to discuss and identify any areas of concern that they may have with their baby. The health care professional will be able to gain valuable information relating to the baby's feeding patterns, sleep patterns, the number of wet and dirty nappies and if the parents have any areas of concern. This will help them greatly in assessing the baby's well-being and (except for feeding patterns which were discussed in Chapter 5) these will all be discussed further below.

Sleep and alert states

Understanding normal sleeping and waking patterns is important for the health care professional. If you understand normal behaviour you will be able to identify when behaviour isn't normal and take appropriate action. Generally babies should initiate feeds, suck well on the breast (or bottle) and they should settle in between feeds. A baby should not be excessively irritable, tense, sleepy or floppy (NICE, 2006).

Soon after birth the baby has a period of alertness in which there is time for interaction between the parents and baby. This usually lasts for about one hour. The baby may then sleep for a few minutes or for several hours. A further period of reactivity often occurs and then there is usually a marked variation in routine but most well babies will awake around the time of a feed. There are a range of sleep states that may be observed and are normal.

- **Deep sleep**. Characteristics of this deep sleep include closed eyes with no movement, regular respiration, response to stimuli delayed and quickly suppressed. Jerky movements may occur at intervals.
- **Light sleep**. Characteristics of this include irregular respiration, sucking movements, intermittent response to stimuli that occurs more rapidly than in a deep sleep, and rapid eye movements may be seen through the closed lids. Babies may have a drowsy state in which there is fluttering of the eyelids, a startle response or a smile may occur and they may have some limb movements.
- **Quiet alert state** is when a baby's motor activity is minimal but the baby is alert to visual and auditory stimulation.
- **Active crying state** is one in which the baby cries vigorously and may be difficult to console.

(Brazelton, 1984; Brazelton and Nugent, 1995)

Colic

Parents may be concerned that their baby is crying too much, particularly in the evenings when it has fed well and doesn't appear to have a reason to be crying. This may be due to colic. Colic has been described as continuous crying when the baby is otherwise healthy and well fed. It usually occurs in the evening. It can be very hard to get the baby to settle. The baby may draw its knees up to its chest and clench its fists (Directgov, 2007). No one really knows why colic can occur but three possible causes are thought to be:

1. trapped wind when the baby swallows air bubbles when feeding;

2. poor digestion because the intestines are immature, and so the baby may get cramps as the milk passes through the intestine;
3. lactose intolerance.

(Directgov, 2007)

The parents may ask for suggestions on how to reduce or cure the colic. You may not be able to cure it but you could offer parents advice such as ensuring they always burp their baby after a feed to prevent the build up of air in the baby's tummy. If the mother is breastfeeding it may be worth her trying to avoid consuming too much coffee and tea or spicy foods. You may need to reassure the parents that colic is very common and, although it may be distressing for the baby and its parents, research shows that babies with colic eat and gain weight normally (Directgov, 2007).

Physiological assessment

Once you have established with the parents that the baby is sleeping and waking appropriately you may wish to undertake a physiological assessment of the baby. When assessing the physical condition, observation is an important tool. Before undertaking any physical assessment of the baby or touching the baby you must wash your hands in order to prevent infection.

Position

Consider how the baby is lying. A healthy full-term baby will lie in a flexed position and will demonstrate unco-ordinated but strong equal movements on both sides. A baby that is 'floppy' (hypotonic) with weak movements may be unwell.

Respiration

Babies undertake diaphragmatic chest and abdominal breathing (respiration). They normally breathe irregularly, the chest should be symmetrical and they should be breathing quietly through their nose. When awake they should give a loud lusty cry. The normal respiratory rate for a healthy term baby is 30–60 breaths per minute (bpm) (NICE, 2006).

Weight

Weight is an important consideration in determining well-being. The average weight of a baby born at term is 3 500 g–3 750 g (Stables and Rankin, 2005). It would be expected and acceptable that a baby may lose up to ten per cent of its birth weight if weighed on the third day after birth, due to water loss following delivery (Coad and Dunstall, 2005). However, by the fifth day it would be expected that a baby would have regained this initial weight loss and returned to its birth weight. Any baby that has lost more than ten per cent of its birth weight on day three, or that has not returned to its birth weight by day five, should be referred for medical advice.

When you are weighing babies it is important to ensure that they are weighed naked and to be aware that slight variations may occur between weighing scales.

Information box 1

Example of calculation for day three for baby Bob

Bob's birth weight	=	3 500 g
10%	=	350 g
Bob's weight at day 3	=	3 100 g
Bob's weight loss	=	400 g

Therefore, Bob's weight loss is more than 10% and should be referred for medical opinion.

Skin assessment

The baby's skin colour is important in determining well-being and, again, it is important that you become familiar with normal skin colours so that you are able to identify significant abnormalities and know when to call for medical help. The baby's colour may depend upon its ethnic origin; however, he or she should be centrally pink. If lips and tongue are pink this is usually a good indicator that the baby is centrally pink. The baby may have blue hands and feet for up to 24 hours after birth. This is known as acrocyanosis and is a normal feature of the baby (Witt, 2003).

Signs of dehydration

Assessment of skin can give important indicators of neonatal well-being. Eyes and mouth should be moist. If the skin is dry, pale and cool to touch this may indicate that the baby is dehydrated. If gently pinched, the skin may be slow to retract. You may find that the baby has sunken fontanelles (see Information box 2) and that its eyes look sunken. The baby may also have a fast heartbeat (tachycardia). If you are concerned that the baby may be dehydrated you will need to go on to discuss with the parents how many wet and dirty nappies their baby is having and assess whether you

Parents are often concerned if their baby becomes jaundiced and you will need to be able to give them a simple explanation as to why it occurs. Therefore, it is important that you understand the physiological processes that occur which lead to physiological jaundice (Figure 6.1).

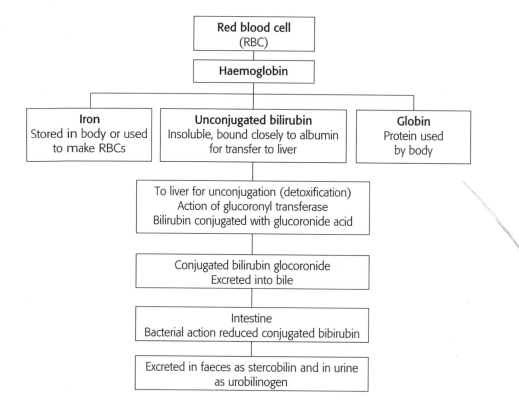

Figure 6.1 Bilirubin breakdown and excretion

When haemoglobin is broken down it is broken down into iron, which is stored in the body or used to make more red blood cells; globin, which is a protein used by the body, and unconjugated bilirubin. Unconjugated bilirubin is toxic. It is fat soluble, cannot be excreted easily in bile or urine and can build up in blood and be deposited in extra vascular fatty and nerve tissues. These deposits under the skin lead to jaundice and deposits in the brain cause bilirubin toxicity and bilirubin encephalopathy (see Chapter 8). In order to travel to the liver to be detoxified this unconjugated bilirubin needs to be bound to albumin for transfer. Once it has been bound to albumin and taken to the liver the action of an enzyme called glucuronyl transferase means that the bilirubin is conjugated with glucuronic acid to form conjugated bilirubin glucuronide. Conjugated bilirubin is non toxic and is water soluble. The conjugated bilirubin glucuronide is excreted into bile where it is taken to the intestine. Once in the intestine bacterial action reduces the conjugated think the baby is feeding adequately. If you are concerned that the baby isn't feeding or passing good amounts of urine and is becoming unwell you will need to refer the baby for medical assistance.

Information box 2

The fontanelle

The fontanelle is where three or more skull bones meet. These are membranous areas sometimes known as soft spots that allow moulding of the head to take place during childbirth. The anterior fontanelle at the front of the skull usually closes when the baby is 12–18 months old. The posterior fontanelle usually closes 2–3 months after birth (Waugh and Grant, 2001).

Jaundice

Jaundice is quite complex so it may be necessary to read this section two or three times until you gain understanding. Yellow skin or jaundice may be a normal feature of the baby skin colour (physiological jaundice). However, it may also be a symptom of underlying disease (pathological jaundice). Jaundice is defined by Percival (2003, p. 863) as 'the yellow discolouration of the skin and sclera that results from raised levels of bilirubin in the blood (hyperbilirubinaemia)'. It is important that the health care practitioner is able to distinguish between physiological (normal) jaundice and jaundice that may be due to an underlying disease (pathological). Within this chapter physiological jaundice will be discussed. The significance of pathological jaundice and its treatment will be discussed in Chapter 8. However, any baby that is born with jaundice or that develops jaundice in the first 24 hours of life should be immediately referred for medical help as this will be a pathological and not physiological jaundice.

Physiological jaundice

Physiological jaundice is a common occurrence in the baby and it is estimated that 50–60 per cent of term babies will become jaundiced (Halamek and Stevenson, 2002). Breastfed infants appear to be more likely to become jaundiced than those fed artificial formula and you may hear the term 'breastfeeding jaundice'. However, Gartner (2001) asserts that breastfeeding jaundice is now regarded as a normal part of physiological jaundice rather than a separate disorder.

bilirubin, which can then be excreted in urine or faeces. The average concentration of serum conjugated bilirubin in babies is 3–7 times higher than that of adults.

There are four reasons why babies are susceptible to physiological jaundice.

1. Increased red blood cell breakdown. To enable the fetus to maximise the carrying of oxygen it has required higher concentrations of erythrocytes (red blood cells). Once born the baby no longer needs this and the baby must change from fetal haemoglobin to adult. Red blood cells in the baby have a short life span (70–90 days instead of the usual 120 days), which means that more red blood cells are being broken down.
2. Reduced levels of albumin. As discussed above, in order to effectively transfer unconjugated bilirubin to the liver it must be bound to albumin. Babies have reduced albumin concentrations (compared with older children). This means that the ability of babies to effectively transfer bilirubin to the liver for conjugation is reduced. There is an increased risk of 'free' unconjugated bilirubin moving back into circulation and going to the skin and brain.
3. Limited production of glucuronyl transferase. The ability of the liver to conjugate bilirubin is reduced because of limited production of glucuronyl transferase and a normal level is not reached until the baby is 6–14 weeks old (Percival, 2003).
4. Increased enterohepatic reabsorption. There is an increased risk of reabsorption from the gastrointestinal tract. This is because babies lack the normal bacteria that reduce bilirubin to urobilinogen. Bowel activity is decreased until feeding is established, which increases the chance of the bilirubin being hydrolysed back into an unconjugated state. Two of the reasons it is thought that breastfed babies are particularly susceptible to physiological jaundice are:
   (a) due to the delayed clearance of meconium; and
   (b) enhanced fat absorption (and absorption of unconjugated bilirubin) from the gut in a breastfed baby.

The assessment of jaundice

Assessment of a baby with jaundice is important. First the health care practitioner needs to decide if this is a baby with physiological or pathological jaundice. As stated above, any baby that is born with jaundice or that develops jaundice in the first 24 hours of life should be immediately referred for medical help as this will be a pathological and not physiological jaundice. Physiological jaundice in a healthy term infant will occur usually around the third day of life (Dhilo, 2005).

To assess how pronounced the jaundice is the health care practitioner needs to use trained eyes; the more babies you assess with jaundice the better you will become at detecting when a level may be high and the baby in need of medical attention. You need to consider where you are looking at the baby. It is important that you are in daylight or a well-lit area as, if you look at a baby in poor lighting or in a room with yellow walls or furnishings, the baby may seem more jaundiced than it is. Some practitioners recommend using 'body zones' in order to assess how high the estimated serum bilirubin (SBR) may be and thus if the baby may be in need of medical attention (see Figure 6.2). If you apply direct pressure to the baby's skin to cause blanching this will allow you to see how pronounced the jaundice is. Therefore, on day three, if the jaundice is only present on the face then the SBR is unlikely to be a cause for concern. However, if jaundice is present in zone 3, 4 or 5 you may need to seek medical opinion, especially if the baby is unwell.

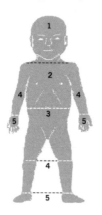

- Zone 1 SBR 100
- Zone 2 SBR 150
- Zone 3 SBR 200
- Zone 4 SBR 250
- Zone 5 SBR >250

(Royal Prince Alfred Hospital, 2006)

Figure 6.2 Body zones for assessment of jaundice
www.cs.nsw.gov.au/rpa/neontal/html/docs/jaundice.rtf

Care of a baby with jaundice

If you are concerned that a baby has significant levels of jaundice you need to consider the care that the baby will need. If the baby is otherwise well, you might advise the parents to undertake some basic care that will help reduce jaundice. This would include ensuring that the baby has regular three- to four-hourly feeds to increase gut motility and diminish the reabsorption of unconjugated bilirubin. Regular feeding will also introduce bacteria to the gut to aid the reduction of bilirubin to urobilinogen. Mothers of a breastfed baby should be encouraged to feed the baby frequently and the baby may need to be wakened to feed (NICE, 2006). Breastfed babies should not routinely be supplemented with formula milk, water or dextrose water (NICE, 2006). You should be aware of and look for signs of any deterioration in the baby's condition that may mean that the baby requires medical attention (NICE, 2006). These signs may include pallor, hypotonia (floppiness), reluctance or refusal to feed, excessive sleepiness, vomiting, high-pitched cry, pyrexia and respiratory distress. Some babies will require phototherapy and this will be discussed in Chapter 8. If jaundice develops after seven days or remains for longer than 14 days in an otherwise healthy baby medical opinion should be sought (NICE, 2006).

Rashes

Skin rashes may be common in the baby, However, most are not significant of illness and are self limiting. It is important that you are able to determine the difference between those which are significant and those which are 'normal'.

Information box 3

Normal rashes

- **Milia** are often seen in babies. They are white or yellow sebaceous cysts that are usually seen on the nose, cheek or sometimes forehead. They are not harmful and usually disappear by the end of the first week of life.
- **Miliaria** (sweat rash) is caused by obstruction of the sweat glands, often because of a warm humid environment. Advise the parents to keep the infant clean and dry.
- **Bruising** of the skin (on the face or scalp) may be a result of a traumatic delivery particularly in forcep or ventouse deliveries. This should disappear within the first week to ten days. Other bruising should be noted (see Chapter 10).
- **Erythema toxicum** is a rash of white or yellow elevated papules that occur on red (erythmatous) skin. The cause is uncertain and this usually resolves itself in a few days. Parents should be advised to keep the skin clean and dry and if you are concerned you should seek medical opinion.

Information box 4

Rashes that may require medical attention

- **Nappy rash.** This can be caused by poor hygiene, infrequent nappy changing, infection or sensitivity to detergents, fabric softeners or other products that may be in contact with the skin. Parents should be advised to change the nappy frequently to ensure the skin is kept clean and dry. A change of detergent to a non-biological product may help in some cases (Michie, 1996). Perfumed creams or wipes should be avoided. If the nappy rash is painful and persistent you should seek medical opinion (NICE, 2006).

- **Thrush.** This is a fungal infection that presents as white spots/patches over the tongue and mucous membranes of the baby. It may be seen as a red rash on the perineum. If thrush is present on the mother's nipples this may be transferred to the baby during breastfeeding and if the baby has thrush in its mouth this may be transferred to the mother's nipple. If the symptoms are causing pain to the woman or baby, or there are feeding difficulties, then you should refer for medical opinion as antifungal treatment may be required (NICE, 2006). Advise the woman to wash and dry her breasts before and after feeding and to avoid the use of perfumed products.
- **Paranychia.** This is redness around the nail bed. It can indicate the presence of an infection and the baby may need medical treatment. You should look at the finger tips and toes to check for this.

Skin care

As well as undertaking assessment of the skin you will be expected to advise parents on appropriate skin care for their baby. Most babies are not bathed immediately after birth to protect skin flora and the baby from infections. This means that babies may be discharged home from hospital without having their first bath. Parents may want reassurance on how to bath their baby. The parents should be advised to ensure that they bath a baby in a warm room with no draughts to ensure the baby doesn't lose heat by convection. Cleansing agents, lotions and medicated wipes for babies are not recommended (NICE, 2006); only a mild non-perfumed soap should be used. Parents should be advised to gather all the equipment together before they start so that the baby doesn't become exposed and cold while parents try to find something. There is no right or wrong time to bath a baby, it is whenever convenient for the parents and when there will be no distractions. You may wish to advise them to switch on the telephone answering machine. Parents should be advised never to leave the baby in the bath unattended. The water should be warm and comfortable for the parents and they should test the temperature of the water before putting the baby in the bath. Women who have had a caesarean section should not be carrying baby baths full of water as this will pull on their weakened abdominal muscles. Once bathed the baby should be quickly dried to prevent heat loss by evaporation and then dressed. It is important to dry carefully in the skin creases because babies may become sore in these areas. Parents may be advised that it is not necessary to bath a baby every day but they need to keep the nappy area clean and dry.

CORD AND EYE CARE

Cord and eye care are also an important area of consideration and parents may be particularly anxious about the care of the cord. Parents should be advised to keep the cord clean and dry. They should be advised that the use of antiseptics is not recommended (NICE, 2006). The area around the cord may be cleaned with warm water. If using disposable nappies they may need to fold down the nappy slightly so that the cord is exposed to enable it to dry. If the skin around the cord becomes inflamed they should seek medical advice as the baby may have an infection and require a course of antibiotics. A swab of the cord should be taken prior to commencing antibiotics. The cord as it dies off may become slightly smelly and sticky. Parents may be reassured that this is normal and to keep the area clean and dry.

Although generally no eye care is needed, sometimes the eyes may become 'sticky'. They may be cleaned using cooled boiled water and a separate clean piece of cotton wool should be used for each eye. The eye should be wiped from the middle out and then the cotton wool discarded. If the eye becomes inflamed and excessively sticky the baby may have an eye infection and may need a swab taken and some eye ointment prescribed by the doctor. Persistent sticky eye may be due to a blocked tear duct and parents should seek advice from the doctor.

NAPPY ASSESSMENT

One of the good indicators of neonatal well-being is how many dirty nappies babies are having and the type and consistency of the bowel motion being passed. Babies should pass stools and urine at regular intervals (NICE, 2006). You would normally expect a baby to have passed urine within 24 hours of birth (Tucker Blackburn, 2003). The kidneys are functionally immature and the capabilities are limited. The urine passed should be dilute, straw coloured and odourless. Initially the term baby will pass 15–60 ml/kg of urine per day in the first few days of life (Tucker Blackburn, 2003). Mucous and urates may be passed by the baby in the urine. This makes the urine cloudy and may be seen as a brown/pink chalky staining in the nappy (Farrell and Sittlington, 2003). Parents may be reassured that this is perfectly normal and nothing to be concerned about.

Pseudomenstruation may be seen as a small amount of red bloodstaining in the nappy of baby girls and is a normal occurrence in the first few days of life. This is due to hormone changes (Cavaliere, 2003).

You would normally expect a healthy term baby to have their bowels open within 24 hours of birth (NICE, 2006). If the baby has not passed a stool you should consider if this is due to poor feeding or a structural abnormality (see Chapter 8). The colour of the stool will change as the baby commences regular feeding. On day one you would expect the stool to be green/black and sticky. This is called meconium and it contains bile salts, fatty acids, mucous, epithelial cells, blood cells, vernix lanugo and secretions from intestinal glands. It has been forming in the fetus from 16 weeks' gestation (Tucker Blackburn, 2003). On day two to three, once the baby has started feeding regularly, you would expect the stool to become green/brown. This is often called the 'changing stool'. By the tenth day the type and frequency of bowel movements will depend upon whether the baby is breast or bottle feeding. A baby who is breastfed will pass loose, bright yellow and inoffensive-smelling acid stools. Often described as like 'mustard seeds'. The baby may pass stools eight to ten times a day or it may pass just one every one to three days (Johnston *et al.*, 2004). For a breastfed baby anything within this range may be normal. For a baby that is artificially feeding the stool will be paler in colour, be semi-formed and have a sharp smell. The baby who is artificially fed will normally pass between four to six stools per day. There is an increased risk of a baby becoming constipated if it is being artificially fed and the health care professional should be aware of this. If you suspect the baby is constipated you will need to tactfully ensure that the parents are preparing feeds according to the manufacturer's instructions, that the baby is taking good amounts of feed and at least four to six hourly (NICE, 2006). If the baby hasn't had their bowels open since birth or you are concerned that they are unwell you should refer the baby for medical opinion.

SAFETY

Safety is an important consideration in ongoing care and it is particularly important for you to identify safety issues, particularly in the home environment. The National Service Framework for Children, Young People and Maternity Services says that all parents should be given information on reducing the risk of sudden infant death and on how to help prevent accidents and non-intentional injury (DH, 2004).

Sudden Infant Death

Perhaps the biggest concern to parents is the risk to their baby of Sudden Infant Death. Sudden Infant Death (SIDS) is 'where a child (usually under the age of one year) dies in their sleep. There is no known medical reason why this happens' (Directgov, 2007). The Department of Health and the Foundation for Sudden Infant Death give parents clear advice on how to help reduce their baby's risk of cot death. As the health care practitioner advising parents it is important that you reiterate this advice. Parents may require reassurance that sudden infant death is rare. Since the introduction of the Foundation of Sudden Infant Death campaign to 'reduce the risk of cot death in 1991' there has been a 75 per cent reduction in the number of sudden infant deaths (FSID, 2007).

Current recommendations are that a baby should be laid on its back to sleep (DH, 2007). The risk of sudden infant death is increased if the baby is in a prone or side-sleeping position (Fleming *et al.*, 1996; Guntheroth and Spiers, 1992). The DH (2007) recommends that babies should be laid on their tummies to play, to help prevent flattening of their heads where they usually lie. Pillows are not recommended for babies under the age of two.

The baby should be placed with feet to the foot of the cot. This will mean that the baby cannot wriggle down under the covers (FSID, 2007). The NICE postnatal guidelines recommend that the use of a dummy is not suddenly stopped (NICE, 2006). The DH (2007) recommend that the baby shares a room with its parents in a crib or a cot for the first six months of life. They go on to recommend that the baby does not share a bed with its parents if either are smokers, have been drinking alcohol, take any drugs or medication that make them sleepy, are exceptionally tired or if the baby was premature, small for gestational age at birth or is under three months old (FSID, 2007). Parents should never sleep with their baby on a sofa or in an armchair as there is a risk the adult may suffocate the baby. If a parent is concerned that a baby is unwell they should seek medical advice promptly (FSID, 2007).

Exposure of babies to smoking by any member of the household before or after birth increases the baby's risk of SIDS (Blair *et al.*, 1996). The DH (2007) recommend that mothers stop smoking during their pregnancy and do not let anyone smoke in the same room as their baby.

Parents are often concerned about the correct temperature for babies; you will need to advise them about appropriate room temperatures and how warm their baby should be. Parents should be advised not to let their baby become too hot and to make sure that while sleeping the baby's head remains uncovered. The recommended temperature for the baby's room is 18°C (65°F) (DH, 2007). All-night heating is rarely required and parents should keep the room at a temperature that is comfortable for them. It is recommended that babies are never left to sleep in direct sunshine, next to a radiator, heater, or a fire, hot water bottle or an electric blanket as these may make the baby too hot. Parents should be advised to remove baby's hats and extra clothing as soon as a baby is brought indoors or into a warm environment even if it means that parents have to wake the baby. In summer the baby may only need a sheet to keep it warm and parents should remember that a folded blanket counts as two blankets.

Parents should be reassured that if a baby's hands or feet feel cool this is normal and not necessarily a sign that the baby is cold. However, if the rest of the body feels cold as well then the baby may need extra clothing or blankets. If the baby is sweating or their tummy is hot to the touch then parents could be advised to take some bedding off the baby to help it to cool down. The baby's temperature in a normal room environment should be 37°C (NICE, 2006).

Calling for medical help

The NICE postnatal guidelines recommend that at each postnatal visit parents are given information that will allow them to assess their baby's general condition, identify common health problems and to know when to call a health professional or emergency help for their baby. The DH (2007) give the following advice for parents and it is important that as health care professionals we are sure that parents know that if their baby demonstrates any of the symptoms below it may be suffering from a serious illness and that they should call for early medical advice.

Information box 5

When to call for medical help
- The baby has a high-pitched or weak cry, is less responsive, much less active than is usual for their baby or is floppy.
- The baby looks pale all over its body, is grunting with each breath or seems to be working hard to breathe.
- The baby takes less than a third of its usual amount of fluids, passes much less urine, has green fluid vomits or has blood when it has its bowels open.
- The baby has a high fever and/or is sweating a lot.

Information box 6

Emergencies (dial 999)

Parents should be advised to call for urgent medical attention (by dialling 999) if their baby displays any of the following:

- stops breathing or goes blue;
- doesn't respond and has no awareness of what is going on around them;
- has eyes that are glazed and don't focus on anything;
- appears to have a fit.

Other safety issues

The health care practitioner should be aware of simple things such as ensuring that a baby is not left on a high surface from where it may be able to wriggle and fall. If the parents are using scratch mittens on their baby they should ensure that they have French seams to ensure that loose threads do not get tied around the baby's finger and thumb and cause a ligature that could occlude the blood supply to the finger or thumb. Care should be taken with animals. There have been a number of high-profile cases of young children being attacked by dangerous dogs and parents should be advised of the dangers of keeping such pets with young children. The use of cat nets may be recommended to prevent the cat from sleeping on the baby. In hospital you should be aware of issues such as ensuring that correct name tags or security tags remain in place until the baby has been discharged by the hospital. Although it is very rare, there have been known cases of strangers making successful and unsuccessful attempts to take babies from postnatal wards. You should ensure that you follow the security measures in your hospital.

Most parents have already bought car seats by the time their baby is due to leave hospital. However, it may be worth noting that children under three years must use a child restraint suitable for their weight in any vehicle. The only exception is in the rear of a taxi if the right child restraint is not available. A rear-facing baby seat should be used for children up to 13 kg (from birth to around 9–12 months). Rear-facing baby seats must not be used in a seat protected by a frontal airbag unless the airbag has been deactivated (Department for Transport, 2006).

NEONATAL VACCINATION AND IMMUNISATION

BCG for Tuberculosis

Most vaccines are given over the baby's first year of life and until recently the immunisation programme didn't commence until the baby was two months old. However, in 2005 the Department of Health (DH) announced changes to the Bacillus Calmette-Guerin (BCG) vaccination programme. This meant that certain babies at high risk of tuberculosis (TB) would be targeted to ensure early vaccination in the neonatal period. Tuberculosis is an infectious disease that usually affects the lungs but it can affect almost any part of the body (DH, 2006a). In the United Kingdom the incidence of TB has been slowly increasing over the past 20 years and about 700 cases are diagnosed in the United Kingdom each year (about 1:10 000 of the population) (DH, 2006a). However, although the number of cases of TB has been rising, the increase has been within specific population groups; hence the Government introduced selective targeted vaccination. Currently any infant under 12 months of age, born or living in areas where the incidence of TB is 40 per 100 000 of the population or greater, should be offered a BCG vaccination (DH, 2005). Previously unvaccinated new immigrants from countries with a high prevalence of TB are also offered the BCG vaccination.

Hepatitis B

In 2005 the British Medical Association (BMA) called for universal immunisation in childhood for Hepatitis B (BMA, 2005). However, the current Government recommendation is that Hepatitis B vaccine should only be given to babies whose mothers or close family members have been infected with Hepatitis B (DH, 2006b). If identified as being at risk the baby should receive the first dose of the Hepatitis B vaccine within two days of birth, the second at one month old, the third at two months old and a booster as well as a blood test at 12 months of age. The vaccine is effective for the majority of babies. Evidence suggests that once the baby has developed immunity it will keep this for life (DH, 2006b).

Key points
- Health professionals must be able to advise parents on the normal behavioural and physiological parameters in their babies.
- Advice should be given about normal sleeping and waking patterns.
- Skin assessment is important to assess for infection and jaundice.
- Safety advice should be given in order to enable parents to provide a safe environment for their babies and to reduce the risk of cot death.

- It is important to have some knowledge of early vaccinations that may be offered.
- If you are unsure, refer to the professional who can give advice or treatment.

Exercises

1. Mother is concerned about baby Billy who has not opened his bowels for two days. He is breastfed. He is sleeping when you visit and his mother says he is producing lots of wet nappies.
   - What other information would you need to gain from her?
   - What advice would you give her?

2. When you visit Sarah her baby Louise is three days old. She weighed 3 800 g at birth and Sarah is worried about her feeding. When you weigh her she is 3 200 g.
   - What other information do you need from Sarah?
   - Has she lost more than 10 per cent of her birth weight?
   - What action will you take?

3. You visit baby Dora on day three. What assessments would you carry out? Her mum is concerned because she has become slightly jaundiced overnight. What explanation and advice will you give to her parents and why?

4. Donna is a smoker and is anxious about sudden infant death. What advice would you give her to help reduce the risk?

5. Dianne is worried that she has not been offered Hepatitis B vaccine for her baby because her friend Jane's baby had this vaccination last week. What would you advise her to do?

REFERENCES

Blair, P.S., Fleming, P. J., Bensley, D., Smith, I., Bacon, C., Taylor, E., Berry, J., Golding, J. and Tripp J. (1996) 'Smoking and the sudden infant death syndrome'. *British Medical Journal*, 313: 195–198

Brazelton, T.B. (1984) *Neonatal Behavioural Assessment Scale* (2nd Ed.). London: Heinemann

Brazelton, T.B. and Nugent, J.K. (1995) *Neonatal Behavioural Assessment Scale* (3rd Ed.). London: McKeith Press

British Medical Association Board of Science and Education (2005) Hepatitis B vaccination in childhood **www.bma.org.uk/ap.nsf/Content/ Hepbchildhood**

Cavaliere, T. (2003) 'Genitourinary Assessment', in Tappero, E. and Honeyfield, M. *Physical Assessment of the Newborn: a comprehensive approach to the art of physical examination* (3rd Ed.). Santa Rosa, CA: NICU INK

Coad, J. with Dunstall, M. (2005) *Anatomy and Physiology for Midwives* (2nd Ed.). Edinburgh: Elsevier Churchill Livingstone

Department of Health (1996) 'Confidential Enquiry into Stillbirths and Deaths in Infancy 1 January–31 December 1994'. London: DH

Department of Health (2004) *National Service Framework for Children, young People and Maternity Services*. London: DH

Department of Health (2005) *Changes to the BCG Vaccination Programme*. London: DH

Department of Health (2006a) *Tuberculosis Factsheet*. London: DH

Department of Health (2006b) *Immunisation for Life*. NHS Immunisation Information. London: DH

Department of Health (2007) *Reduce the risk of cot death: an easy guide*. London: DH

Department for Transport (2006) Law: Use the right car seat for your child. **www.thinkroadsafety.gov.uk**

Dhilo, E. (2005) 'Neonatal Jaundice', in Thureen, P., Deacon, J., Hernandez, J. and Hall, D. *Assessment and Care of the Well Newborn*. Philadelphia: Elsevier

Directgov (2007) Colic and jaundice. **www.direct.gov.uk/en/Parents/ HavingABaby/After TheBirth/DG_10039685**

Farrell, P. and Sittlington, N. (2003) 'The Normal Baby', in Fraser, D. and Myles, M. (eds) *Myles Textbook for Midwives* (14th Ed.). Edinburgh: Churchill Livingstone

Fleming, P.J., Blair, P.S., Bacon, C., Bensley, D., Smith, I., Taylor, E., Berry, J., Golding, J. and Tripp, J. (1996) 'Environment of infant during sleep and risk of sudden infant death; results of 1993–5 case-control study for confidential enquiry into stillbirths and deaths in infancy'. *British Medical Journal*, 313: 191–195

Foundation for Sudden Infant Death (2007) **www.fsid.org.uk/babycare. html**

Gartner, l. (2001) 'Breastfeeding and Jaundice'. *Journal of Perinatology*, 21: S25–S29

Guntheroth, M.D. and Spiers, P.S. (1992) 'Sleeping prone and the risk of sudden infant death syndrome'. *Journal of the American Medical Association*, 267: 2359–2362

Halamek, L. and Stevenson, P. (2002) 'Neonatal jaundice and liver disease', in Fanaroff and A. Martin, R. (eds) *Neonatal-perinatal Medicine: Diseases of fetus and infant* (7th Ed.). St Louis: Mosby

Johnston, P., Flood, K. and Spinks, K. (2004) *The Newborn Child* (9th Ed.) Edinburgh: Churchill Livingstone

Michie, M. (1996) 'A delicate concern: caring for neonatal skin'. *British Medical Journal*, 4 (3): 159–163

National Institute for Health and Clinical Excellence (2006) *Routine post-natal care of women and their babies*. London: NICE

Nursing and Midwifery Council (2004) *Midwives rules and standards*. London: NMC

Percival, P. (2003) 'Jaundice and infection' in Fraser, D. and Cooper, M. (Eds) *Myles Textbook for Midwives* (14th Ed.). Edinburgh: Churchill Livingstone

Royal Prince Alfred Hospital (2006) 'Neonatal jaundice', in *RPA Newborn Care Protocol Book*. Camperdown: RPA. **www.cs.nsw.gov.au/ rpa/neonatal/html/docs/jaundice.rtf**

Stables, D. and Rankin, J. (2005) *Physiology in Childbearing with Anatomy and Related Biosciences* (2nd Ed.). London: Elsevier

Tucker Blackburn, S. (2003) *Maternal, Fetal and Neonatal Physiology: A Clinical Perspective* (2nd Ed.). Philadelphia: W.B. Saunders

Waugh, A. and Grant, A. (2001) *Ross and Wilson Anatomy and Physiology in Health and Illness* (9th Ed.). Edinburgh: Churchill Livingstone.

Witt, C. (2003) 'Skin assessment', in Tappero, E. and Honeyfield, M. *Physical Assessment of the Newborn: a comprehensive approach to the art of physical examination* (3rd Ed.). Santa Rosa, CA: NICU INK.

Useful Websites

www.cry-sis.org.uk

www.dh.gov.uk/en/Publicationsandstatistics/Publications/
PublicationsPolicyAndGuidance/DH_4123625

www.nice.org.uk

Chapter 7

Communication
Karen Bates

Chapter aims

To explore aspects of communication to ensure effective transition to parenthood.

Learning outcomes
By the end of this chapter you will be able to:

- discuss the psychological transition to parenthood and the midwife or nurse's role in facilitating this transition;
- demonstrate an understanding of how to support parents who have a neonate requiring extra care;
- describe the factors that may influence psychological health;
- describe the importance of the role of debriefing after delivery, the role of voluntary organisations and the importance of interprofessional/interagency collaboration in supporting families.

Mapping to standards of proficiency

Standards of Proficiency for Pre-registration Midwifery Education (SPME)
Communicate effectively with women and their families throughout the preconception, antenatal, intrapartum and postnatal periods, listening to women, jointly identifying their feelings and anxieties about their pregnancies, the birth and the related changes to themselves and their lives.
Enabling women to think through their feelings.
Enabling women to make informed choices about their health and health care.
Actively encouraging women to think about their own health and the health of their babies and families, and how this can be improved.
Communicating with women throughout their pregnancy, labour and the period following birth.

Standards of Proficiency for Pre-registration Nursing Education
Provide support and education in the development and/or maintenance of independent living skills.

Engage in developing and disengaging from therapeutic relationships through the use of appropriate communication and interpersonal skills.
Identify and respond to patients' and clients' continuing learning and care needs.

NHS Knowledge and Skills Framework (NHS KSF)
Core 1, Level 2
Communicate with people on a range of matters.
The worker:

- communicates with a range of people on a range of matters in a form that is appropriate to them and the situation;
- improves the effectiveness of communication through the use of communication skills;
- constructively manages barriers to effective communication;
- keeps accurate and complete records consistent with legislation policies and procedures;
- communicates in a manner that is consistent with relevant legislation, policies and procedures.

INTRODUCTION

This chapter does not profess to include everything that has been written, and is known about, effective communication between a health care professional and client. The aim of this chapter is to explore factors that underpin communicative episodes so that the health care practitioner may be better placed to facilitate a more effective transition to parenthood for the women they are caring for.

The bedrock of health care is effective communication. Good communication with a woman and her family can be the key which unlocks the mysteries of surviving the early days of being a new parent; a time that has been referred to as 'the crisis of parenthood' (McCourt, 2006). Health care practitioners who communicate well are more likely to secure positive outcomes for their clients and themselves (Berry, 2007). In its simplest terms, a positive outcome will be one where a message has been received and understood. The purpose of the message will determine the subsequent action.

Helping women to make choices during pregnancy and in the early days with a new baby is about more than just telling them information. Women need to understand the information in order to make their choices. Effective communication is the means by which information that will be fundamental to the women making informed decisions is imparted (DH, 2004; Berry, 2007). Women worry about feeding, crying babies, sleeping patterns, developmental milestones and successful bonding. The list is endless and also very personal, differing between one woman and another and between one parent and another in the same family. Unless the health care practitioner is able to communicate skilfully, how can she plan care which is appropriate and responsive to individual need?

When health care practitioners communicate with parents, the act of communication is simply the observable behaviour, the tip of the iceberg. Underneath the surface the process of delivering and receiving a message will be affected by a number of covert factors (Sully and Dallas, 2005). This chapter will begin by providing some generally accepted principles of good practice in relation to communication. It will go on to look at the meaning of motherhood. Raphael-Leff's (2005) seminal work will be considered as one way by which a health care practitioner may understand why a woman is reacting to motherhood in the way that she is. It will go on to examine the psychological factors that underpin communication as well as attitudes to successful parenting and how these may impact on the communicative episodes.

It will consider the changes that need to be made during the transition period from being a childless couple to becoming parents, and how a health care practitioner can facilitate this transition period. It will demonstrate how a failure to recognise these central, implicit factors can create psychological barriers to effective care. No assumptions are made in this chapter as to the variance in the meaning of 'couples' or 'parents'. It is acknowledged that these concepts are multifaceted in twenty-first-century Western Europe. For ease of purpose this chapter will use these terms to mean a man and woman, married or unmarried, in a stable relationship. However, there are principles of understanding that can be applied to anyone becoming a parent either as a sole parent or in a less conventional relationship.

The principles of caring for women during the transition period are applicable to all women. However, the chapter will also consider what additional support may be needed when the newborn baby requires extra care.

GENERAL PRINCIPLES FOR EFFECTIVE COMMUNICATION

Communication is a sharing of facts, information, attitudes and feelings. Very often in health care we recognise the facts and information side of communication as there is a wealth of facts and information we are expected to impart to women and receive from women. Less awareness or consideration is given to the other less explicit side of communication, but even before the health care practitioner opens their mouth to communicate facts and information, they have communicated attitudes and feelings which will impact on the way the message is received by the other person.

A linear model of communication has evolved from the very early attempts at defining a model of communication and includes the following (Figure 7.1):

Source → encoder → message → channel → decoder → receiver

Figure 7.1 Model of communication

The following shows how this linear model of communication can be applied to a scenario of a health care practitioner who is initiating a communicative episode with a woman (adapted from Sully and Dallas, 2005; Hargie and Dickson, 2004).

Source

The health care practitioner becomes the source. They may be consciously aware that they are initiating a communicative episode because they have information to share, or they may not be aware that they are the source of communicating a message because it is not a verbal message, it is non-verbal and implied in their body language.

Encoder

The health care practitioner organises the message into a physical form capable of being transmitted. In a face-to-face communicative episode this becomes the mouth and voice box and would not be something the practitioner is aware of. It may also be a collection of articles or leaflets; or the arranging of an interpreter to attend, who will be better placed to encode the message into a language the woman can understand.

Message

The message is the content of the communicative episode. This can be not only whatever the practitioner wants to share, but also the hidden message that the practitioner does not want to send, for example, the non-verbal communication. Problems occur when the verbal, conscious communication does not match up with the non-verbal, subconscious communication. Consideration needs to be given to the complexity of the message. Is it information that needs to be imparted? If so, how best may this be achieved? Sometimes information given during the postnatal period can be complicated and requires understanding so that a woman may reach an important decision involving not just herself but also her new baby. Written information is useful as an aid to the verbal explanation that accompanies it. Written information should not be used as a replacement for the verbal explanation. All too often a written leaflet is considered the panacea to the problem of the health care professional not having time to sit and talk with the woman.

Channel

The channel can be considered the means by which the source (i.e. the health care practitioner) and the receiver (i.e. the woman) are connected. It can be further broken down into:

- **vocal-auditory** – a channel that carries speech, for example, the telephone, sound waves, etc.;
- **gestural-visual** – a channel that facilitates non-verbal communication, for example, face-to-face communication, television, etc.;
- **chemical-olfactory** – a channel that accommodates smell, for example, interpersonal contact.
- **cutaneous-tactile** – a channel that facilitates use of touch, for example, interpersonal contact and face-to-face communication.

(from Hargie and Dickson, 2004)

An update to this list would include electronic methods for sending messages such as e.mail. These channels are used more and more in society as a means of sending a message.

Decoder

The decoder is the system or structure which makes sense of the message. In a face-to-face communicative episode between health care practitioner and woman, the decoding system is the ear, decoding the sound waves into vibrations that are carried along the auditory nerve to the brain, which decodes it further into language. If it is non-verbal communication that is being decoded, it is the eye and brain that become the systems for decoding the message in the same way. In a communication by e.mail it is the computer system that organises the message into a form that will be understood by the receiver.

Receiver

The receiver is the person for whom the message is intended and who will make sense of it. The way someone makes sense of a message will be very individual and dependent on their own personal attitudes, beliefs, expectations and how they are feeling at any one moment. Almost as soon as the message is received, the receiver becomes the sender of another message which is a response, so a health care practitioner can be the source and receiver within the same communicative episode.

The above model is the most simplistic of the models of communication, but it can provide the practitioner with a framework that enables them to understand why they find themselves in a situation where they have been misunderstood. They have sent a message that they believe to be innocent or without any particular 'other' meaning, but it is misinterpreted by the other person who reads some hidden meaning behind the message. By using this model they can check back to each part of the communicative episode and determine which element may have been a possible cause or reason for the misunderstanding.

MOTHERHOOD

Childbearing has been described as a phase in the life cycle of the family (Raphael-Leff, 2005). The arrival of the first child represents a major transition in a person's life (Weiten, 2004). Becoming a mother means taking on a new identity, which involves a complete rethinking and redefining of self (Mercer cited in Bryar, 1995; McCourt, 2006; Ball, 1994). To progress from being nulliparous to primiparous (non-mother to mother) or from being primiparous to multiparous (mother of one to mother of others) changes a woman's relationships, her body, her identity, her behaviour and her future (Nicholson, 1998; Smith, 1999). Motherhood is a challenge – hard work and stressful – but this is not to say that it doesn't bring with it immeasurable rewards. The way an individual will take on this changing role will be influenced by their own reactions, largely defined by their personality and the responses between themselves and the people around them including family, their child and 'others', i.e. the health care professional (Ball, 1994).

We know from Jean Ball's seminal work on the postnatal period that the way women respond emotionally to the birth of their baby will be affected by their own personality and the quality of support received from other family members and social support systems, including midwives. On the one hand this is an intensely personal experience; on the other it is very public. 'Motherhood' is a prescribed social role and the processes involved in the childbearing period are reinforced and validated by 'experts' – midwives and doctors (Nicholson, 1998). The implications are that, without even being aware and conscious of it, messages about what is 'good mothering' can be communicated to the women at this vulnerable time in their lives.

In her book *Psychological Processes of Childbearing*, Joan Raphael-Leff (2005) discusses changes that need to be made at an emotional level when making the transition to parenthood. Her psychoanalytical approach to this area of practice provides a style, or orientation, that women may fit into.

Information box 1

Facilitator
- Relishes pregnancy and natural childbirth.
- Postnatally she adapts to her baby.
- Her life is centred around her new baby.

Regulator
- Strives to control aspects of the pregnancy.
- Does not want to lose her self-control during labour.
- Expects her baby to adapt to her and aims to regulate the baby.

Reciprocators
- Accepts and tolerates ambiguity and uncertainty.
- Does not approach childbirth and the postnatal period with ingrained expectations.

There is a fourth group and this is considered to be the 'extreme' group or 'conflicted group'. This group will exhibit pathological reactions which spill over into the rest of the family (from Raphael-Leff, 2005: U4).

The Facilitator will have been preparing for the moment when she becomes a mother. She is 'tuned in to' this baby and this role. The kind of behaviour a Facilitator may exhibit in the postnatal period would be that of a woman who expects to breastfeed, to be a full-time carer, to have close proximity to her baby, and to be exclusively devoted to her baby's needs – both physical and emotional.

Conversely, the term 'confinement' would aptly suit the way a Regulator views pregnancy and motherhood. Rather than tuning in to the baby's needs as the Facilitator would do, it is more a case of her expecting the baby to become tuned in to the family. She may be the type of woman who is heard to say her life will not change with the arrival of the new baby, and the skiing holiday will still be booked. She will rationalise that it makes little difference to the baby who undertakes childcare and will have little concern about returning to work with good childcare systems in place.

Such challenges will be handled differently by Facilitators. For example, financial constraints may leave a woman with little choice but to go out to work which, for a Facilitator, is going to create tensions as she will be forced to be a different kind of mother from the kind she expected to be. The key to making the transition less stressful may be to have realistic expectations about what it means to be a parent (Belsky and Kelly, 1994; Weiten, 2004).

At a time when the majority of parents are enjoying their new babies and exploring them, showing them to visiting family and friends, there will be a small number of babies admitted to a neonatal unit. Parents of these babies not only have to cope with the stresses of childbirth, they now find themselves in a situation where their hopes and expectations of having a normal experience and a healthy baby at the end are not realised (Lindsay and Meehan, 1994). The mother must deal with the physical effects of childbirth, and both parents have to cope with this highly technological, frightening environment, which becomes the bittersweet giver and taker. On the one hand, it gives their baby the best chance of survival with its bleeping machines and monitors which alarm. On the other hand it has taken their baby away from their bedside, their arms and their family; even temporarily, this is a loss to the new parents. Applying Raphael-Leff's model to this scenario, we can visualise the Facilitator unable to have the close proximity to her baby that she craves and which is some-thing fundamental to her sense of fulfilment in being a mother. The Regulator's sense of order and clearly defined expectations will have been thrown into chaos.

A health care practitioner who is consciously or unconsciously competent (Howell, 1982) will be aware of the distress of the new parents in this situation and the impact of this alarming environment and will apply interventions and strategies as appropriate. This type of practitioner will be better able to reach women at the emotional level and be more effective in responding to the psychological needs of the new parent. Parents of a baby admitted to a neonatal unit and thus separated from them during the early days following delivery, need to have the fear taken out of the monitors that alarm and the machines that bleep, by having the equipment explained to them. The health care practitioner becomes the conduit between parents and machines, through which the parents are given back some control and understanding. Parents can be encouraged to touch their newborn baby, to see past the incubator and be confident that this relationship with their baby will be satisfactory in fostering the embryonic development of the baby's sense of self. Women need to know and understand that a baby has no sense of 'self' and cannot distinguish between themselves and any other person or object. The fact that the baby is separated from the mother will not mean the relationship will for ever be flawed. Part of the maturing process is the creation of a sense of self and an awareness of internal boundaries.

Even if the health care practitioner does not have anything particularly concrete to offer in terms of further advice, parents may just appreciate feeling that the professional is 'involved' in what they say or that they are being listened to (Brown *et al.*, 2006).

In applying the Facilitator/Regulator framework there is a danger of over-simplifying the situation and making a generalisation that all women will respond to circumstances in one of these two ways. Practitioners know that not all women will fit nicely into one or other of these categories and, indeed, the women may fit different categories at different times in their lives. The question that is sometimes asked of me by students trying to get to grips with the application of this theory to practice is, 'So how useful is it?' My answer is that it provides a framework for beginning to anticipate and prepare for the myriad of responses women exhibit to pregnancy and being a mother. What it does enable is a deeper insight into our own emotional responses to the way a mother may react, especially if her reaction is at odds with our own personal values or attitudes.

Jean Ball's research examined how women react to motherhood (1994). Her study concluded that reactions to becoming a mother are complex and determined by a myriad of factors; some internal factors such as personality, particularly for highly anxious women, and some external factors such as the environment.

Early motherhood is a time of intense emotional responses. Health care practitioners need to be 'with woman' during this period as much as at any other period during the pregnancy and birth. They need to be able to respond to the new mother and her emotions without judgement. How we view women as mothers and our own sense of self will influence our professional relationships and, as health care practitioners, we may move closer to being able to understand why a woman behaves in the way she does when she becomes a mother.

FACTORS UNDERPINNING COMMUNICATION

Every interaction between a health care practitioner and the client will be preceded by personal history. What is being said in the here and now cannot be divorced from each person's personal conscious and subconscious experiences. How people interrelate and interpret experiences is grounded in their cultural and personal heritage (Sully and Dallas, 2005). Communication between health care practitioners and the person accessing the service is recognised as a very complex process that moves beyond being a simple 'sender–receiver' model of communication (Brown *et al.*, 2006).

Let us consider the scenario of a healthy baby, being seen by the midwife during the early postnatal period. The midwife or maternity care assistant must undertake care within certain parameters. This care includes weighing the baby, neonatal screening tests, making sure the baby is physically fit and healthy and feeding well. It is important that these factors are monitored. However, the parents may have other concerns. For the Regulator, it may be how soon she can wean her newborn baby so she may return to work but, if she admits this to the health care practitioner, would she be viewed as a bad mother because she should be maintaining breastfeeding for as long as possible in the postnatal period? For the Facilitator it may be that, in spite of all her preparation and certainty that she will tune in to her new baby, the reality is different. In spite of her best efforts, she is unable to decipher her baby's crying signals and she feels she is failing.

Both women in these scenarios may well be worrying about what the health care practitioners think of her – will they think she is a 'bad mother'? Women watch for every attitude displayed by a professional.

Concepts of parenting

Is there such a concept as successful or unsuccessful parenting, which impacts on our attitude to women in the postnatal period? Each one of us will have ingrained in our psyche our own personal schema of parenting and will attribute to this schema the additional dimension of success or failure. Schemas are personal cognitive structures that help individuals to process information (Weiten, 2004). A person will use a schema to organise the world around them (Weiten, 2004; Sternberg, 2004). Some of the schema people hold about parenting and being a parent will be unique to their own personal experiences. Every parent is a parent of their own child and the child of their own parents. Other schema may also be part of a shared cultural background (Weiten, 2004).

Overlaying this construct will then be the attribution of success or failure. Theorists have explained the attributions people make in explaining success and failure as being due to either internal factors or personal attributions, or to external factors or situational attributions (Weiner, cited in Weiten, 2004; Heider, cited in Sternberg, 2004). Attribution theories help us to explain our own behaviour and the behaviour of others (Sternberg, 2004). As a Western consumer society we are bombarded with images of so-called 'good' parenting. Many parents see anything less than expensive, top of the range, mix and match baby accessories as not good enough. Could this be the shared cultural 'norm' shaping our view of what is a successful parent?

Attitudes are evaluative (Weiten, 2004). In other words, humans will internalise information, judge it in terms of their own personal value systems and experiences and make an evaluation. The evaluation will be positive or negative and can be attributed to objects or thoughts. Occasionally a person may hold both positive and negative attitudes about something. This is known in psychological terms as an ambivalent attitude.

Psychologists have suggested that attitudes may comprise up to three components (see Figure 7.2):

- the cognitive component – the beliefs people hold about an object or thought;
- the affective component – the emotional feelings stimulated by an object or thought;
- the behavioural component – predispositions to act or behave in a certain way.

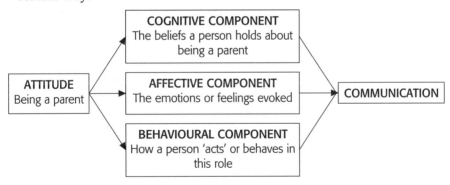

Figure 7.2 Diagrammatic representation showing the link between attitude and communication

The implicit assumption here will be that we are aware of the attitude we may hold about something. We can use frameworks and models of communication to help us to understand our own attitudes and feelings about parenthood, in order to begin to recognise the covert issues that may impact on our verbal and non-verbal communication skills. Johari's window (Figure 7.3) was created in the 1950s by Joseph Luft and Harry Ingham. It is a tool that may provide a practitioner with insight as to how they communicate with others but, equally importantly, they may gain some idea of how others perceive them.

	Known to self	Not known to self
Known to others	**Open**	**Blind spot**
Not known to others	**Hidden**	**Unknown**

Figure 7.3 Communicating with others

This model is particularly useful for practitioners who need to address deep-seated feelings about circumstances that are affecting the way they are able to respond to women and their needs. Take, for example, the issue of termination of pregnancy. This subject can evoke very strong personal feelings, which affect the observable response. A practitioner may have very deep-seated feelings and opinions about termination of pregnancy as being fundamentally wrong. The practitioner may have no problems with vocalising these feelings to other people and the feelings then become 'open' – i.e. they are known to the practitioner and to other people.

Within the 'hidden' window we may find that the practitioner experienced a termination of pregnancy early in her life, which she deeply regrets and has clearly not been able to come to terms with. The practitioner will know this, but other people will not. The 'blind spot' for the practitioner may be that what other people are observing is quite an aggressive, abrupt way of dealing with women who are attending hospital for termination of pregnancy, particularly if they appear to be quite blasé about it. The practitioner herself is not aware of the way she is behaving to these women; she is blind to it.

The 'unknown' window will decrease in size depending on the level of underpinning knowledge and understanding that each party has. If the practitioner herself can begin to understand the effect of her previous experience on her behaviour in the here and now, she will be better able to put plans in place to deal with it and less will be unknown to her. The more that is understood by the other people, the more able they will be to move closer to understanding why the practitioner is behaving in the way she is and they may be better placed to help her.

There is a dearth of information and guidance for health care practitioners about pregnant women with disabilities and their experiences of motherhood (McGuiness 2006; McKay-Moffat and Cunningham, 2006). This lack of knowledge and understanding about caring for women with disabilities has an impact on how effectively such women's needs are discussed. In particular, midwives were found to be worried about saying the wrong thing for fear of insulting or upsetting the women (McKay-Moffat and Cunningham, 2006). There can be a lack of liaison with other health care professionals in order to seek support and advice, and this adds to any already existing communication problem.

CONCLUSION

This chapter has explored some factors which underpin communication. It has not been an exhaustive exploration; that would not be possible. Hopefully, it has raised enough enquiries in the reader's mind as to the importance of considering underlying factors that have an effect on the tiny part of observable behaviour, which in turn affects the quality of communication. It is only by considering these underlying factors that practitioners can begin to address the real needs of women and not what 'we' perceive them to be.

Key points
- The meaning of motherhood is different for every individual.
- Maternity carers must examine their own attitudes to the meaning of motherhood.
- It is perfectly normal to have a deeply ingrained sense of what makes a good mother or a bad mother. The problem lies with not recognising this personal emotional response. Without recognising it, communication is affected; it becomes a 'blind spot' to us. Worse still, no one in the health care system recognises any sort of communication problem, indicating that problems are deeper than the individual and permeate the structure of the service.

Exercises

1. You are working on an early shift on a busy postnatal ward. You are asked to provide care to a postnatal woman on her third day. As you enter her room, you see she is on the verge of tears and her baby is crying. If you applied Raphael-Leff's model to this woman, she could be categorised as a Facilitator.

   - How will you initiate communication with this woman?
   - How will you ensure that communication has been effective?
   - How does the application of Raphael-Leff's framework enable you to assess her needs and determine a plan of care for her?
   - How might this care plan look if this were a 'Regulator'?

2. You are working on the Special Care Baby Unit and looking after a seven-day-old baby. His mother has visited twice since she was discharged. She is a young parent who is clearly finding the transition to motherhood, with the accompanying responsibility, difficult to cope with. When she visits, she does not stay for very long and rushes off to be with her friends. Applying the attitude model above:

   - How would you determine your attitude to this young woman and the way she is with her baby?
   - How might this attitude affect your approach to this woman?

3. Using Johari's window above (Figure 7.3), reflect on a time when you were trying to communicate with another person (it may have been a woman, a member of her family or another health care practitioner). It may have been about a particularly sensitive situation, for example, talking a woman through her decision to have a termination of pregnancy, talking to a woman about her decision to bottle feed her baby, or talking to a senior midwife or obstetrician about a woman or baby you may have been concerned about and they did not share the same concerns.

REFERENCES

Ball, J. (1994) *Reactions to Motherhood: the role of postnatal care.* Cambridge: Cambridge University Press

Belsky, J. and Kelly, J. (1994) *The Transition to Parenthood.* New York: Dell

Berry, D. (2007) *Health Communication Theory and Practice.* UK: Open University Press

Brown, B., Crawford, P. and Carter, R. (2006) *Evidence-Based Health Communication*. UK: Open University Press

Bryar, R. M. (1995) *Theory for Midwifery Practice*. UK: Palgrave

Department of Health (2004) *National Service Framework for Children, Young People and Maternity Services*. London: Department of Health

Hargie, O. and Dickson, D. (2004) *Skilled Interpersonal Communication*. UK: Routledge

Howell, W. (1982) *The Empathic Communicator*. Wadsworth: Pacific Grove

Lindsay, B. and Meehan, H. (1994) *The Child and Family*. UK: Balliere Tindall

McCourt, C. (2006) 'Becoming a Parent', in Page, L., McCandlish, R. *The New Midwifery*. UK: Churchill Livingstone

McGuinness, F. (2006) (Editorial) 'Effective communication is the core of effective practice'. *British Journal of Midwifery*, 14 (8): 452

McKay-Moffat, S. and Cunningham, C. (2006) 'Services for women with disabilities: mothers' and midwives' experiences'. *British Journal of Midwifery*, 14 (8): 452

Nicholson, P. (1998) *Postnatal Depression: Psychology, science and the transition to motherhood*. London: Routledge

Raphael-Leff, J. (2005) *Psychological Processes of Childbearing* (4th Ed.). UK: Anna Freud Centre

Smith, J.A. (1999) 'Identity Development during Transition to Motherhood: an interpretive phenomenological analysis'. *Journal of reproductive and infant psychology*, 17 (3): 215–235

Sternberg, R. J. (2004) *Psychology*. UK: Thomson

Sully, P. and Dallas, J. (2005) *Essential Communication Skills for Nursing*. UK: Elsevier

Weiten, W. (2004) *Psychology: Themes and Variations* (6th Ed.). UK: Thomson

Chapter 8

Neonatal Disorders
Julie Mullett and Amanda Williamson

Chapter aims

To enable you to competently recognise a neonate with special needs and initiate appropriate care for the neonate.

Learning outcomes

By the end of this chapter you will be able to:

- identify the neonate who has special needs, this will include: prematurity, small for gestational age, hypoglycaemia, pathological jaundice, infection, cardiac anomalies;
- discuss the appropriate actions for the health care practitioner to undertake in this situation.

Mapping to standards of proficiency

Standards of Proficiency for Pre-registration Midwifery Education (SPME)
Effective Midwifery Practice
Examine and care for babies with specific health or social needs and refer to other professionals or agencies as appropriate.
This will include:

- low birth weight
- pathological conditions (such as babies with vertical transmission of HIV, drug-affected babies).

Standards of Proficiency for Pre-registration Nursing Education
Manage the delivery of care services within the sphere of one's own accountability.
Consult other health care professionals when individual or group needs fall outside the scope of nursing practice.
Establish priorities for care based on individual or group needs.
Demonstrate the safe application of the skills required to meet the needs of patients and clients within the current sphere of practice.
Recognise the need for adaptation and adapt nursing practice to meet varying and unpredictable circumstances.

INTRODUCTION

This chapter will explore common disorders that may occur in the baby during the postnatal period. The health care practitioner will need to know how to recognise and take appropriate action should these problems occur. This chapter will initially discuss the care of the well premature and small for gestational age baby. It will go on to discuss the recognition of, and the health care practitioner's role in, caring for babies with hypo-glycaemia, pathological jaundice, infection and congenital heart disorders.

The main emphasis of this textbook has been to examine the health care practitioner's role in caring for the normal term baby. It is essential, however, that the health care practitioner has an understanding of their role in the identification of common disorders that may occur in the newborn baby; and of their role in caring for a baby who is under the care of the neonatologist or paediatrician. The chapter will build upon the definitions of neonates as outlined in Chapter 1.

PREMATURE/SMALL FOR GESTATIONAL AGE BABIES

Premature and small for gestational age babies (defined in Chapter 1) may, depending upon the degree of prematurity or birth weight, be admitted to the hospital's neonatal unit directly from the delivery suite following delivery. Many units, however, will care for moderately prema-ture babies (those born between 35 to 37 weeks of pregnancy) and babies defined as low birth weight (2 500 g or less) (see Chapter 1) within a transitional care environment. You may find in your role as health care practitioner you are allocated to look after these babies either within special care of a neonatal unit, within a transitional care setting or on the postnatal wards. It is therefore essential that you are aware of the unique needs of these babies and their parents.

Temperature control

Although delivery rooms are kept relatively warm, the ideal room temperature being 25°C (Rutter, 2005, p. 272), the baby, once delivered, will start to lose body heat immediately. This is lost through the four processes of conduction, convection, evaporation and radiation (see Chapter 3). If you are present at a delivery where the baby is small for its gestational age, or premature, it is important that you assist in ensuring the baby is kept warm and dry, as a baby weighing 1 kg can lose 1°C for every five minutes they are exposed (Rutter, 2005).

The main source of heat production for the newborn baby is through metabolic activity (feeding) (Rutter, 2005). The newborn baby is capable of producing heat to try and maintain their body temperature in response to being cold. They do this through non-shivering thermogenesis and, to some degree, through vasoconstriction of peripheral blood vessels. Non-shivering thermogenesis is the production of heat through the metabolism of brown fat. Newborn premature babies have virtually no ability to produce heat through shivering and, unlike the term infant that can to some degree move into a flexed position to try and conserve some heat, the preterm baby is limited in their ability to do this. Most preterm babies will lie in their cot or incubator in a flaccid relaxed position, which leaves much of their skin exposed and vulnerable to heat loss.

It is important for the baby to maintain a stable body temperature to ensure growth and maintenance of energy needs. The aim of the health care practitioner is to ensure that the baby is kept adequately warm to make sure that a thermoneutral state is achieved. This is when the baby is in a state of minimal energy expenditure and oxygen consumption in order to maintain a normal body temperature of 37°C (NICE, 2006).

Maintenance of a thermoneutral state is more difficult to achieve in the premature and small for gestational age baby. Due to the large body surface area relative to body weight, the premature baby and small for gestational age baby have a greater capacity to lose heat than the term and appropriate for gestational age baby. The premature and small for gestational age baby has fewer fat stores (Lucas and Fewtrell, 2005) to insulate them from heat losses and depleted stores of brown fat and glucose. They are therefore limited in their ability to generate heat. If the baby requires admission to the neonatal unit, they may need to be initially cared for in an incubator. You should refer to your local guideline for the admission criteria to the neonatal unit. As the baby matures the temperature of the incubator can be lowered. However, initially a premature or small for gestational age baby weighing 2.0–2.5 kg admitted to special care who needs an incubator will need the incubator to be set at approximately 32°C–34°C (Rutter, 2005). While the baby is cared for in the incubator you will need to monitor their temperature regularly as overheating can also affect the baby by causing fluid loss (Yeo, 1998). Some neonatal units will dress well babies while they are still cared for in the incubator but you will need to refer to your local guideline regarding this. However, if you do dress the baby, you will need to remember to reduce the temperature of the incubator accordingly.

A premature or small for gestational baby on a postnatal or transitional care ward will require regular monitoring of their temperature. You will need to refer to your local guidelines for exactly how often to record the baby's temperature. However, once stable, this is usually undertaken three to four hourly, along with feeds and nappy changes. To maintain a normal temperature these babies may require additional clothing. This is best achieved through layering of clothes such as a vest, sleepsuit and cardigan. You need to be aware that these small babies lose most of their heat through their head and often require a hat to keep warm (Rutter, 2005). If the baby becomes cold or is cold on admission, one method of achieving a normal body temperature is through the use of a radiant heater. Most hospitals will have a mobile radiant heater to warm babies and you will need to refer to your local guidelines on which babies this is most appropriate for and how to use the heater. When using a radiant heater to warm a cold baby you should remember that babies tend to warm very quickly so it is essential that you closely monitor the baby's temperature when using this method. If you use a radiant heater to warm a cold baby it is often better to remove the baby's clothing as this will ensure the baby reaches a normal body temperature much more quickly. It is also good practice to warm the baby's clothes under the heater so that you are able to dress the baby in warm clothes once they have reached a normal body temperature. This, in turn, helps to reduce the risk of further heat loss by conduction. The same principles for ensuring the baby doesn't lose heat by convection apply as discussed in Chapter 3, i.e. shutting doors and windows to prevent draughts.

Feeding

The aim of nutritional support in the postnatal period is to provide enough for the baby to achieve optimal growth. The method used to provide nutritional support to the premature and small for gestational age baby will ultimately depend upon the baby's gestational age, weight and condition. Very small, premature or sick babies may require their nutritional support to be provided initially by an intravenous infusion of either dextrose or total parental nutrition with the introduction of oral feeds being delayed until the baby is either older or more stable. The ultimate aim of feeding is to introduce full oral intermittent milk feeds via breast or bottle. This may, however, need to be introduced in the more premature baby with minimal milk feeds at first, increasing slowly to full oral feeds only as feeds are tolerated.

The health care practitioner needs to be aware that the ability to suck and swallow is a reflex action that only becomes evident in the premature baby at approximately 34–35 weeks gestation (Lucas and Fewtrell, 2005). Prior to this the baby, if able to tolerate oral feeds, may require them to be administered either by naso-gastric tube or by cup feeding. Even when the baby reaches this gestation the majority of premature and small for gestational age babies become tired easily and are not able to take all their feeds via bottle or breast. You will need to be aware of your local trust guideline in relation to the introduction of feeds but most hospitals will introduce regular three- to four-hourly feeds, slowly increasing not only the volume each day as tolerated by the baby but also the amount taken via bottle or breast. These babies are at increased risk of hypoglycaemia (low blood sugar) and this is discussed further below.

Hypoglycaemia

Glucose homeostasis (normal glucose regulation)

Blood glucose needs to be maintained within a narrow range and the pancreatic hormones insulin and glucagon are central to this. Most organs are able to cope with short periods with reduced levels of glucose. However, glucose is essential for the baby's brain to function effectively (Johnston et al., 2004). Insulin and glucagon are secreted by the islet cells that are scattered throughout the pancreas. They secrete hormones into the bloodstream. This enables them to gain access to cells far away and make those cells respond in a particular fashion.

Insulin

Insulin is secreted by the beta islet cells. As blood glucose increases the amount of insulin secreted rises and as blood glucose falls the amount of insulin secreted also falls. In response to insulin, cells absorb glucose from the blood, thus lowering blood glucose.

Glucagon

Glucagon is secreted by the alpha cells of the pancreatic islet cells. If the blood glucose is high no glucagon is secreted and if the blood glucose is low more glucagon is secreted. Glucagon has an effect on many of the body cells but most notably on the liver. The effect of glucagon on the liver is to make it release more glucose into the bloodstream. Blood glucose concentration levels are detected by the pancreas. Therefore, a high blood glucose leads to increased insulin production and a corresponding decrease in glucagon. The glucose is converted to glycogen and stored in the liver, and blood glucose is lowered.

Adaptation to extrauterine life

Glucose is the major substrate for carbohydrate metabolism in newborn babies as, after birth, the baby loses its source of glucose from its mother. Falling plasma insulin levels and slow production of insulin prevent glucose being taken up by cells. An increase in serum glucagon levels mobilises glucose from intracellular glycogen stores. Liver glycogen stores decrease rapidly as 90 per cent is utilised in the first 24 hours after birth and muscle glycogen reduces by 50–80 per cent (Tucker Blackburn, 2003).

Hypoglycaemia

Hypoglycaemia is the commonest metabolic abnormality in infancy (Cornblath *et al.*, 2000). It most commonly occurs when the normal processes of metabolic adaptation after birth fail to occur. The baby must meet two major metabolic challenges. The baby needs to maintain adequate circulatory concentrations of glucose or alternative fuels to supply the body's organs. The baby also needs to adapt to a new form of intermittent nutrition (Tucker Blackburn, 2003).

There are various definitions of hypoglycaemia and no clear consensus of what an acceptable level of blood glucose in babies is (Tucker Blackburn, 2003). However, in general it may be best defined as blood glucose of below 2.6 mmols/l (WHO, 1997).

Information box 1

Reasons for hypoglycaemia in a baby. It may be due to:

- Depleted or limited glycogen stores. Babies in this category would include:
  -- small for gestational age babies;
  -- premature babies;
  -- a baby who has an infection;
  -- a baby who has hypothermia or has been hypothermic (had a low temperature);
  -- a baby with a rare metabolic disorder such as glycogen storage disorder (Johnston *et al.*, 2004);
  -- a baby who has been hypoxic (low levels of oxygen) before birth or has had birth asphyxia;
  -- twins because they are likely to be smaller than a single pregnancy, or the second twin may have suffered some hypoxia before delivery;
  -- babies who have a congenital cardiac disease.

- Hyperinsulinaemia (high levels of insulin). Babies in this category would include:
  -- a baby of a diabetic mother (Johnston *et al.*, 2004);
  -- a baby with Beckweith-Weiderman Syndrome;
  -- a baby whose mother had a dextrose infusion prior to delivery.

You will need to be alert to the signs and symptoms of a baby who may have hypoglycaemia (see Information box 2 below) and call for early medical help as hypoglycaemia may lead to convulsions and has implications for long-term neurodevelopment outcomes (Hoseth *et al.*, 2000). However, the most important thing as a health care practitioner is that you are able to take action to prevent hypoglycaemia occurring.

Prevention of hypoglycaemia

To prevent hypoglycaemia the health care practitioner must identify those babies at risk (see above). It is important that you prevent the baby becoming cold. This is perhaps the most important thing the health care practitioner can do to prevent a baby becoming hypoglycaemic (see Chapter 3). If the baby becomes hypothermic it will use up valuable stores of glucagon. You should also ensure that any baby you have identified as being at risk of hypoglycaemia has early and regular feeds. You should continue to feed the baby with regular (one-, two- or three-hourly) feeds as this will help the baby become used to intermittent feeding. You should also either undertake monitoring of blood glucose for those babies at risk of hypoglycaemia or ask someone to monitor the blood sugar for you. If the baby is unwell or unable to tolerate milk feeds you will need to ask for medical help. You should be aware of the local trust guideline in relation to managing hypoglycaemia in the neonate.

Management of hypoglycaemia

Despite identifying and actively managing those babies at risk, some babies will still develop hypoglycaemia. As said above, the health care practitioner must know the signs and symptoms of hypoglycaemia as it is essential that early treatment be instigated. The health care practitioner should also be aware of the local trust guidelines for the prevention and treatment of hypoglycaemia. Once it has been identified that the baby is hypoglycaemic the management will include correction of the hypoglycaemia and establishment of the cause.

Information box 2

Signs and symptoms of hypoglycaemia may include:

- blood sugar level <2.6 mmol/l (WHO, 1997);
- asymptomatic (no symptoms);
- jitteriness and/or tremors;
- hypotonia (floppy);
- irritability;
- poor feeding;
- tachypnoea (fast breathing);
- abnormal cry, which may be high-pitched or weak;
- unstable temperature;
- convulsions (fitting);
- apnoea (not breathing).

(Armentrout, 2004)

Pathological jaundice

Jaundice is a yellow discolouration of the baby skin and is often described as being either physiological or pathological in origin. Pathological jaundice is jaundice as a result of some underlying disease process. Before continuing with this chapter you may benefit from reviewing physiological jaundice as discussed in Chapter 6.

Information box 3

Pathological jaundice is jaundice which:

- occurs within the first 24 hours;
- is associated with other illnesses;
- is associated with high levels of bilirubin;
- is prolonged >10 days at term and >14 days preterm.

(Mupanemunda and Watkinson, 2005)

It is important that you are able to recognise and understand pathological jaundice as early referral to medical care is essential. Any baby that becomes jaundiced within the first 24 hours of life must be referred immediately for medical help. It is important that you are aware of pathological jaundice as it is very likely that the first person to be alerted to the baby's jaundice will be the health care practitioner undertaking their routine examination of the baby.

It is essential that the health care practitioner is able to recognise those babies at risk of pathological jaundice as high levels of bilirubin (hyperbilirubinaemia) not bound to albumin (see Chapter 6) are easily able to cross the blood–brain barrier and enter into the brain cells causing kernicterus or bilirubin encephalopathy. Bilirubin encephalopathy is characterised by the yellow staining of brain tissue. Although there is no set blood level of bilirubin at which bilirubin encephalopathy is said to occur (Thureen *et al.*, 2005), you should be aware of the importance of seeking medical help if you are concerned about any baby with jaundice. Bilirubin encephalopathy is associated with adverse neurodevelopmental outcomes such as fits, deafness and cerebral palsy and, left untreated, may even result in death (Mupanemunda and Watkinson, 2005).

Information box 4

There are several risk factors that can increase a baby's risk of developing bilirubin encephalopathy. Those at risk are babies who:

- are premature;
- have an infection;
- have had a low blood sugar (hypoglycaemia);
- are unwell.

(Stephenson, 2000)

Information box 5

Common causes of pathological jaundice
- Problems that can cause increased red blood cell breakdown such as infection or excessive bruising.
- Haemolytic disease of the newborn (excessive destruction of the baby's red blood cells) can be caused by a number of blood group incompatibilities.
- Biliary Tract Obstruction which causes abnormal bilirubin excretion.
- Problems that interfere with bilirubin conjugation (detoxification), for example, hypothyroidism or certain drug interactions.

(Kenner and Lott, 2004)

Treatment of jaundice

The aim of jaundice treatment is to prevent the levels of the toxic unconjugated bilirubin in the blood rising to levels that may cause long-term damage. For pathological jaundice phototherapy is always required. It is also important to follow the principles of care outlined in Chapter 6.

Phototherapy works by detoxifing the bilirubin and facilitating its excretion from the body via routes other than by conjugation in the liver. There are a number of methods of delivering phototherapy and you should be familiar with the guidance for the methods used by your Trust. Generally the baby will need to be nursed while exposed under the phototherapy light as the phototherapy will only work on the areas of skin exposed to the light. This means that when caring for a baby under phototherapy there are a number of things you will need to consider. You will need to ensure that the baby is able to maintain its temperature within a normal range. You will need to take actions to ensure the baby doesn't lose heat by evaporation, convection, conduction and radiation (see Chapter 3). It is good practice to cover the baby's eyes to protect them while they are under the phototherapy light (Johnston *et al.*, 2004). The method used to cover baby's eyes will differ depending upon the practices of the Trust you work in, so it is important that you are aware of these.

As the phototherapy works by converting the bilirubin into a form the body is able to excrete, you will find the baby will pass increasing amounts of urine and stools. This means you will need to take extra care of the baby's nappy area, ensuring the baby remains clean and dry at all times. This is especially important if the baby is nursed completely naked under the phototherapy light. As long as the phototherapy is controlling the bilirubin level, medical staff may state that it is reasonable for phototherapy to be interrupted for feeds and parental visits (Mupanemunda and Watkinson, 2005). Some babies will become unsettled when nursed naked under the phototherapy light and may benefit from you making some boundaries in the cot or incubator.

Infection

Newborn babies are susceptible to infection due to the immaturity of their immune responses and their vulnerability to certain infections that can be acquired *in utero* from the mother. The baby may acquire infections during the antenatal, intrapartum or postnatal periods. The fetus is protected *in utero* by the amniotic sac. However, some microorganisms are able to cross the placental barrier. Premature babies have a greater risk of sepsis due to their poorer immunity to infection. Antibiotics are used widely in neonatology and increasingly in obstetrics but this may lead to the obliteration of colonising flora and may increase the risk of super infections. The health care practitioner needs to be aware of the importance of good cord, mouth and skin care in reducing the risk of infection. The baby has some defences to infection and these may be specific or non specific.

Information box 6

Non-specific defences:

- skin – forming a barrier to invading organisms, but any cuts or abrasions, mucosal injury or canulae will increase the risk of bacterial invasion;
- phagocytosis by macrophages and inflammatory responses (Horns, 2004).

Specific defences:

- transfer of immunoglobulin IgG, from the third month of pregnancy – this gives the baby limited immunity to infectious diseases for which the mother has antibodies (Cant and Gennery, 2005).

Immunoglobulin IgA does cross the placenta and is synthesised by babies only after birth. This is present in high concentration in maternal colostrum and breast milk (Fewtrell and Lucas, 2005).

Immunoglobulin IgM is a larger molecule that does not cross the placenta and is responsible for combating infections such as E.coli. IgM synthesis starts in the fetus from approximately 20 weeks and by term has only reached about 10 per cent of the level in adults. If a baby is infected at birth it will have a high level of IgM present in its blood.

Clinical presentation and assessment of the baby with an infection

Although infections may be caused by a variety of micro-organisms there are often many common principles relating to the presentation of infection in babies. Early recognition, diagnosis and treatment of serious infections are essential because the baby's condition can deteriorate very rapidly. It is important that the health care practitioner is able to recognise an unwell baby early to ensure rapid referral to medical help. The health care practitioner needs to be aware that early clinical signs may be subtle and they should have a low threshold for referral, as early treatment is essential for a good outcome.

You should consider if there are any events in the maternal, antenatal or postnatal history that may indicate that this baby may be at a greater risk of infection. If there are any risk factors you should monitor the baby very closely and refer to medical help if the baby shows any signs of becoming unwell.

Information box 7

Risk factors to consider that may lead to infection in a baby
- Was the mother pyrexial during labour?
- Did the mother have any vaginal discharge or a tender uterus during labour that may indicate chorioamnionitis?
- Did the mother have prolonged rupture of membranes? (Percival, 2003)
- Has the mother had any known infectious disease in pregnancy or been in contact with anyone with an infectious disease such as chickenpox?
- Were there any potential infectious lesions on her cervix or in her vagina?
- Consider also if there are any cuts or abrasions on the baby's skin which could act as a portal of entry on the baby for infection.

Information box 8

Signs and symptoms of infection in a baby may include:
- 'Going off' – hard to define but often the earliest and most important sign, often the mother may comment that her baby isn't right.
- Respiratory (breathing) signs – grunting, tachypneoa (fast breathing), chest recession cyanosis (blueness), apnoea (not breathing) (Horns, 2004). Mild respiratory distress of a raised breathing rate (normal rate 30–60 breaths per minute (NICE, 2006)) and slight chest recession are among the first non-specific signs of infection.
- Temperature changes – a temperature raised above 38°C (NICE, 2006) or hypothermia (low temperature) (Horns, 2004).
- Cardiovascular signs – a heart rate greater than 160 beats per minute may be present (NICE, 2006).
- Gastrointestinal signs – the baby may feed poorly, vomit and/or have diarrhoea (Horns, 2004).
- Skin – a raised papular 'pinpoint' rash may be present in an infant with listeria infection (Dear, 2005).
- Central nervous system – the baby may be lethargic, irritable, may have a bulging fontanelle, high pitched cry, seizures (fits) (Horns, 2004).

The health care practitioner needs to be aware that babies with infection may present initially with very subtle symptoms of infection. It is unlikely that an infected baby will present with all the symptoms listed. However, the health care practitioner needs to be aware that any deterioration in a baby's condition after the first two or three days should immediately make you suspicious of an infection. Medical help should always be sought.

Cardiac (heart) disorders

Cardiac disorders that may present in the baby include: structural congenital heart disease; a malformation of the heart or large blood vessels near the heart that is present at birth; acquired heart diseases such as endocarditis (an inflammation of the endocardium and heart valves) and metabolic disorders which involve the heart muscle and may also produce symptoms of cardiac problems in the newborn period.

Congenital heart defects are the most common congenital abnormality the health care practitioner will see in the newborn period (Stephenson, 2000). The government's heart statistics (see **www.heartstats.org**) reports the incidence of congenital heart defects as 6.9 per every 1 000 live births per year. The health care practitioner may already be aware that the baby has a congenital heart defect as approximately 50 per cent of babies born with a congenital heart defect will have been diagnosed antenatally through routine antenatal ultrasound scanning (Stephenson, 2004).

Information box 9

Risk factors associated with congenital heart disease
- Chromosomal abnormalities – several chromosomal abnormalities are also often associated with congenital heart defects such as Trisomy 21 or Down's syndrome and Turner's syndrome (Sadowski, 2004).
- Exposure of the fetus during pregnancy to certain viruses such as rubella (German measles) (Vargo, 2003).

Maternal risk factors include:

- maternal diabetes, systemic lupus erythematosus (Sadowski, 2004).
- maternal congenital heart defect or a brother or sister with a congenital heart defect increases the risk of the baby being born with a congenital heart defect (Park 2002);
- maternal drug use, both prescribed and non prescribed;
- alcohol misuse (Sadowski, 2004).

Care of the baby with congenital heart disease

Care of the baby with congenital heart disease requires the health care practitioner to carefully assess the baby for signs and symptoms that may indicate the presence of a congenital heart defect. If the health care practitioner suspects congenital heart disease they must refer the baby for medical help immediately.

Many congenital heart defects do not compromise the fetus *in utero* as it is reliant upon fetal circulation and the baby doesn't necessarily show any symptoms in the initial postnatal period as it is continuing to adapt to extrauterine life (see Chapter 3 for fetal circulation and adaptation to extrauterine life). It is only as the baby's circulation completely changes from fetal to adult circulation and the ductus arteriosis closes, which occurs at approximately 60 hours of age (Archer, 2005), that significant congenital heart defects may become evident.

> **Information box 10**
>
> **Signs and symptoms of congenital heart disease**
> - Central cyanosis – a blue or bluish discolouration of the skin and mucus membranes that can worsen when the baby cries (Sadowski, 2004).
> - Increased breathing rate.
> - Pallor and mottling of the skin (pale skin colour).
> - Alteration of feeding pattern or poor feeding.
> - Oedema (swelling) is associated with congenital heart disease on rare occasions (Vargo, 2003).

The health care practitioner needs to be able to distinguish central cyanosis from normal acrocyanosis. Acrocyanosis is the blue discolouration of the baby's extremities (hands and feet) that is common following birth and for the first 48 hours and is due to a reduced blood flow through the small capillaries (Rennie, 2005). Acrocyanosis, unlike central cyanosis, only involves the baby's hands and feet and usually resolves within the first few days of life, though it may reappear if the baby becomes cold. If the health care practitioner suspects the baby has a central cyanosis (blue discolouration of the lips and mucous membranes in the mouth are a good indicator of central cyanosis) they should call for immediate medical help.

The health care practitioner also needs to be aware that not all congenital heart defects present with central cyanosis. This means that you should be alert to all signs of congenital heart disease and not rely on the basis that the baby will be blue or cyanosed. Congenital heart defects are often defined as those which present with cyanosis and those which do not.

For further information on structural congenital heart defects and how individual defects present refer to the British Heart Foundation **www.bhf.org.uk**.

As with many of the common disorders that can occur in babies in the newborn period, symptoms of congenital heart disease can often be subtle initially and may not include all the symptoms listed. If you suspect the baby is unwell you must refer the baby for medical help even if you are unsure of the reason.

SUMMARY

This chapter has discussed the care of the well premature and small for gestational age baby, the recognition of, and the health care practitioner's role in caring for, babies with hypoglycaemia, pathological jaundice, infection and congenital heart disorders. As discussed in earlier chapters, it is important that you learn to 'baby watch' as the more you learn to recognise a baby that is well, the sooner you will be able to identify when a baby may be giving subtle signs of becoming unwell. The recognition of these subtle signs will enable you to undertake prompt and vital care actions when caring for babies who have special needs.

Key points
- Well premature and small for gestational age babies may be cared for on the postnatal ward, transitional care ward or within the special care area of a neonatal unit.
- It is important to keep premature and small for gestational age babies' temperatures and blood sugars within normal limits.
- The health care practitioner must be alert to the subtle signs a baby may give if it is becoming unwell and call for early medical aid.

Exercises

1. The paediatrician has just reviewed baby Thomas who is four hours old. Baby Thomas looks jaundiced and the paediatrician has asked you to start phototherapy. Is baby Thomas's jaundice physiological or pathological? What are the possible causes of baby Thomas's jaundice?
2. Baby Leanne is two days old. Her mother informs you that she is not feeding well and feels hot. You take her temperature which is reading 38°C. Why is baby Leanne susceptible to infection? What non-specific defences does baby Leanne have to protect her from infection? What are your immediate actions?

3. Baby Samantha has just been admitted to the postnatal ward at 36 weeks' gestation. You take her temperature as she feels cold and it is recorded as 35°C. By which four processes could baby Samantha have lost heat? What actions will you take to raise Samantha's temperature?

REFERENCES

Archer, N. (2005) 'Cardiovascular disease', in Rennie, J. (Ed.) *Roberton's Textbook of Neonatology*. Edinburgh: Elsevier Churchill and Livingstone

Armentrout, D. (2004) 'Glucose Management', in Verklan, T. and Walden, M. *Core Curriculum for Neonatal Intensive Care Nursing* (3rd Ed.). Philadelphia: Elselvier Saunders

British Association of Perinatal Medicine (2001) *Standards for Hospitals Providing Neonatal Intensive and High Dependency Care*. (2nd Ed.) and *Catagories of Babies Requiring Neonatal Care*. London: BAPM

Cant, A. and Gennery, A. (2005). 'Neonatal infection', in Rennie J. (Ed.) *Roberton's Textbook of Neonatology*. Edinburgh: Elsevier Churchill and Livingstone

Cornblath, M., Hawdon, J., Williams, A., Aynsley Green, A., Ward Platt, M., Schwartz, R. and Kalhan, S. (2000) 'Controversies Regarding Definition of Neonatal Hypoglycaemia: Suggested Operational Thresholds'. *Pediatrics*, 105 (5): 1141–1145

Dear, P. (2005) 'Infection in the newborn', in Rennie, J. (Ed.) *Roberton's Textbook of Neonatology*. Edinburgh: Elsevier Churchill and Livingstone

Fewtrell, M. and Lucas, A. (2005) 'Feeding the full term baby', in Rennie, J. (Ed.) *Roberton's Textbook of Neonatology*. Edinburgh: Elsevier Churchill and Livingstone

Horns, K. (2004) 'Immunology and infectious disease', in Verklan, T. and Walden, M. (2004) *Core Curriculum for Neonatal intensive Care Nursing*. (3rd Ed.). Philadelphia: Elselvier Saunders

Hoseth, E., Jorgensen, A., Ebbesen, F. and Moeller, M. (2000) 'Blood glucose levels in a population of healthy, breast fed, term infants of appropriate size for gestational age'. *Archive of Disease in Childhood, Fetal Neonatal Edition*, 83: 117–119

Johnston, P., Flood, K. and Spinks, K. (2004) *The Newborn Child* (9th Ed.). Edinburgh: Churchill Livingstone

Kenner, C. and Lott, J. (2004) *Neonatal Nursing Handbook*. Philadelphia: Saunders

Lucas, A. and Fewtrell, M. (2005) 'Feeding low birthweight infants', in Rennie, J. (Ed.) *Roberton's Textbook of Neonatology*. Edinburgh: Elsevier Churchill and Livingstone

Mupanemunda, R. and Watkinson, M. (2005) *Key Topics in Neonatology* (2nd Ed.). London: Taylor and Francis

National Institute for Health and Clinical Excellence (2006) *Routine postnatal care of women and their babies*. London: NICE

Park, M.K. (2002) *Pediatric Cardiology for Practitioners* (4th Ed.). St Louis: Mosby

Percival, P. (2003) 'The healthy low birthweight baby', in Fraser, D. and Cooper, M. *Myles Textbook for Midwives* (14th Ed.). Edinburgh: Churchill Livingstone

Rennie, J. (2005) *Roberton's Textbook of Neonatology*. Edinburgh: Elsevier Churchill and Livingstone

Rutter, N. (2005) 'Temperature control and disorders', in Rennie, J. (Ed.) *Roberton's Textbook of Neonatology*. Edinburgh: Elsevier Churchill and Livingstone

Sadowski, S. (2004) 'Cardiovascular Disorders', in Verklan, T. and Walden, M. (2004) *Core Curriculum for Neonatal Intensive Care Nursing* (3rd Ed.). Philadelphia: Elselvier Saunders

Stephenson, T., Marlow, N., Watkins, S. and Grant, J. (2000) *Pocket Neonatology*. Edinburgh: Churchill Livingstone

Thureen, P., Deacon, J., Hernandez, J., Hall, D. (2005) *Assessment and Care of the Well Newborn* (2nd Ed.). Philadelphia: Elsevier Saunders

Tucker Blackburn, S. (2003) *Maternal Fetal and Neonatal Physiology* (2nd Ed.). Philadelphia: Saunders

World Health Organization (1997) *Hypoglycaemia of the Newborn. Review of the Literature*. Geneva: World Health Organization

Vargo, L. (2003) 'Cardiovascular Assessment', in Tappero, E. and Honeyfield, M.E. *Physical Assessment of the Newborn: A comprehensive approach to the art of physical examination* (3rd Ed.). Santa Rosa, CA: NICU INK

Yeo, H. (1998) *Nursing the Neonate*. Oxford: Blackwell Science

Chapter 9

Multiculturalism: Culturally Sensitive Care for the Baby

Nicki Young

Chapter aims

- To provide an introduction to the knowledge required when planning culturally sensitive care.
- To demonstrate the influence that culture, ethnicity and religion may have upon attitudes towards care of the baby.
- To develop practice that promotes the rights, interests, preferences and beliefs of the individual.

Learning outcomes

By the end of this chapter you will be able to:

- recognise the potential influence culture and religion may have upon attitudes towards care;
- demonstrate knowledge to draw upon when planning culturally sensitive care for mothers and babies from diverse backgrounds;
- identify practice that promotes individual rights, interests, preferences, beliefs and cultures;
- reflect upon the principles of health care in a multicultural context in order to provide culturally sensitive and equitable care for all users of the health services.

Mapping to Standards of Proficiency

Standards of Proficiency for Pre-registration Midwifery Education (SPME)
Effective Midwifery Practice
Determine and provide programmes of care and support for women which are appropriate to the needs, contexts, culture and choices of the women, babies and their families.
Practise in a way which respects, promotes and supports individuals' rights, interests, preferences, beliefs and cultures. This will include:

- offering culturally-sensitive family planning advice;
- ensuring that women's labour is consistent with their religious and cultural beliefs and preferences;
- acknowledgement of the roles and relationships in families, dependent upon religious and cultural beliefs, preferences and experiences.

Standards of Proficiency for Pre-registration Nursing Education
Maintain, support and acknowledge the rights of individuals or groups in the health care setting.
Act to ensure that the rights of individuals and groups are not compromised and
Respect the values, customs and beliefs of individuals and groups.
Provide care which demonstrates sensitivity to the diversity of patients and clients.

NHS Knowledge and Skills Framework (NHS KSF)
Core 6, Level 2
The worker:
a) recognises the importance of people's rights and acts in accordance with legislation, policies and procedures;
b) acts in ways that:
   acknowledge and recognise people's expressed beliefs, preferences and choices;
   respect diversity;
   value people as individuals;
c) takes account of own behaviour and its effect on others;
d) identifies and takes action when own or others' behaviour undermines equality and diversity.

INTRODUCTION

The population of the United Kingdom (UK) is increasingly diverse in relation to cultural, ethnic and religious differences (Helman, 2006). Consequently, health care practitioners are likely to care for babies and families from a range of backgrounds. Every family will have a 'culture' and in order to truly provide care that is family-centred and culturally sensitive, the health care practitioner must be prepared to appreciate the needs of the family in terms of culture, ethnicity and religion. Previous chapters in this book have discussed how health care practitioners assess neonatal well-being and much of this assessment rests upon effective communication between the health care practitioner and the parent/parents. Misunderstandings can occur if the health care practitioner does not deliver care that takes account of the needs or wishes of the parents, as interventions may be planned that are not acceptable.

This chapter is divided into four parts. It begins with setting the context for the provision of culturally sensitive health care. The second part discusses culture, ethnicity, race and religion and presents a brief overview of the population of the UK. The next part describes some of the practices that exist around care of the baby; it is not a definitive list but is intended to be an introduction to the existence of difference and diversity in care. The last part contains exercises and questions to prompt your critical thinking and problem-solving by placing you in the role of the practitioner caring for the baby.

BACKGROUND

The provision of accessible and culturally sensitive care to National Health Service (NHS) users is a government priority. The *National Services Framework for Children, Young People and Maternity Services* (NSF) (Department of Health (DH), 2004) firmly establishes that health providers need to be responsive to the diversity and difference which exists in the population served.

The Nursing and Midwifery Council (NMC) *The Code: standards of conduct, performance and ethics for nurses and midwives* (2008) sets out the principles by which nurses and midwives should practise and relate to the general public. One way to meet the principles of the Code is for the health practitioner to gain an understanding of the concepts of culture, ethnicity and race.

EXPLORATION OF CONCEPTS

Culture

Culture is a complex, abstract concept and has been defined by MacLachlan (2006, p. 11) as

> a set of guidelines – a formula – for living in the world...social cultures nurture the growth of people with particular beliefs, values, habits, etc. But, above all, culture provides a means of communication with those around us...culture is the medium through which communication takes place.

As the child grows up he or she will inherit this set of guidelines from the family. The child will assimilate aspects of culture by observing interactions between family members and will be guided in how to behave at family and wider social occasions such as: playing games, birthdays, festivals, religious events, marriages, illness and death. The child will learn how to behave in relation to other people and how to experience the world emotionally. They will learn the rules and meanings inherent in situations that govern daily practices (MacLachlan, 2006).

Every individual has a 'culture', which includes a certain set of beliefs about the customs and traditions that should accompany birth and care of the baby. Cultural influences may change over time and with personal experiences such as: education, occupation and migration. There is great diversity within cultures and great diversity across cultures (Schott and Henley, 1996).

Ethnicity

Ethnicity is not a straightforward concept to define, having many different elements. One way of thinking about ethnicity is that it is a quality

> that refers to the group to which people belong, and/or are perceived to belong, as a result of certain shared characteristics, including geographical and ancestral origins, but particularly cultural traditions and languages.
>
> (Bhopal, 2004, p. 413)

Another way of thinking about ethnicity is that it describes those characteristics of a group of people that provide the group with common markers or a sense of belonging. These markers or characteristics include: language, food, religion, customs, the clothes that are worn, lifestyle and geographical origin (Spencer, 2000). Ethnicity is not fixed and as individuals adapt socially and culturally ethnicity may change.

Race

Historically race was conceived as a biological concept and linked to physical attributes. Over time this argument has been discredited and nowadays the concept of race is seen as being socially constructed, although recognition is given to the fact that the terms 'race' and 'racism' are present in everyday language (Sookhoo, 2003). While in the United States it is more common to use the combined term race/ethnicity, in Europe the term 'race' is being replaced by the term ethnicity (Bhopal, 2004).

Religion

Throughout the world there are many religions. Examples of 'nine major world faiths include: Baha'I, Buddhism, Christianity, Hinduism, Jainism, Judaism, Islam, Sikhism and Zoroastrianism' (Department of Health, 2003, p. 5). However, great diversity exists within these religions and consequently great diversity will exist in the way individuals follow and express their faith. For example, in the Jewish faith there are Orthodox,

Reform and Liberal Jews, each 'group will attend their own synagogues and follow their own traditions' (Schott and Henley, 1996, p. 329).

For some individuals their faith is central to their being and every aspect of daily living revolves around it. For others, religion is not important and will not have any role in their life. Despite this, when faced with birth, illness or death, individuals may turn to religion or their spiritual beliefs as a way to make sense of what is happening to their baby and family unit.

Brief overview of the UK population

Over time the population of the UK has changed, mainly due to the long history of migration into and out of the country. The Office for National Statistics (ONS) is the Government agency responsible for compiling the UK's social and demographic statistics, including the periodic census of the population. The last census of 2001 showed that the minority ethnic population had grown from 3 million in 1991 to 4.6 million. The minority ethnic population accounted for 7.9 per cent of the total population, of which the largest proportion, comprising around a half, were described as Asians of Indian, Pakistani, Bangladeshi or other Asian origin. The next largest category was described as Black; that is Black Caribbean, Black African or Other Black. The remaining minority groups included the Chinese and other ethnic group categories (ONS, 2001). More recently immigration has included citizens from the eight Central and Eastern European countries that joined the Economic Union in May 2004 (ONS, 2007).

Information about the geographical distribution of minority groups shows that, in comparison to the population as a whole, ethnic minorities tend to live in major urban areas or relatively large towns. However, immigrants from Eastern Europe are more evenly distributed across the country and some are now looking for work in areas of the country that traditionally had little or no history of foreign newcomers (ONS, 2007).

PRACTICES SURROUNDING CARE OF THE BABY

It is important when reading the next part of the chapter to bear in mind that great diversity exists across groups and within groups. This means that what one individual wants may be different from what another wants, even if they belong to the same religious, cultural or ethnic group. Schott and Henley (1996) stress that it is very easy to stereotype groups and individuals and the very best way to find out what parents want for their baby is to ask them. Never make assumptions about people or groups.

Beliefs surrounding health and illness

Throughout the world different cultures ascribe different meanings to the concepts of health and illness, which leads people to hold different belief systems about their bodies, diseases and treatments (MacLachlan, 2006). Health and illness may be constructed in terms of the relationship between the human and spirit world. In the West the professional health sector has become dominated by scientific medicine and the biomedical model of care. In contrast, many other countries and cultures have long-standing influential systems of medicine, with their own ways of diagnosis, intervention and treatments. For example, the Ayurvedic traditional system of medicine is found in the Indian subcontinent and is over 2000 years old and Chinese medicine has been practised for centuries. Many parents may not be familiar with the technology associated with a hospital or a special care baby unit and they may also be unfamiliar with the screening and surveillance which accompanies care of the baby (Sookhoo, 2003). This means that health care practitioners need to be tolerant of other explanations for illness and disease even though they may not correspond to their own belief system.

Practices surrounding the birth of the baby

In the West it has become common practice at the birth for the baby to be placed onto the mother's abdomen for skin-to-skin contact, or the baby may be given to the mother or partner to hold immediately. In some cultures bodily secretions are believed to be unclean, so the baby needs to be washed to remove blood and vernix, before either parent will hold or feed the baby.

In the Jewish religion restrictions apply to women who are bleeding from the uterus. The woman and her partner are not allowed to touch each other or pass objects between themselves, which includes the baby. This restriction will also prevent close physical contact between the mother and partner at the birth (Schott and Henley, 1996).

Welcoming ceremonies

Specific ceremonies may need to be conducted at the birth of the baby to welcome the baby into the faith. In Hinduism the symbol Om, which means supreme spirit, may be written with honey or ghee on the baby's tongue.

In the Islamic faith the father or a respected member of the community whispers the Adhan or Call to Prayer into the baby's ear (Holland and Hogg, 2001). This also fulfils the requirement that the first sound a child hears will be from a Muslim. Another ceremony may be performed where a piece of date or honey is rubbed into the baby's upper palate. According to Sheikh and Gatrad (2001) the positive attributes of the person performing the ceremony will be transferred to the baby. Muslim babies may be given a symbolic amulet called a *taweez* which is a piece of thread or threads that may contain a small prayer pouch and is placed around the baby's wrist (Sheikh and Gatrad, 2001).

Gender

Finding out the sex of the baby is usually important to parents regardless of culture. Schott and Henley (1996) discuss the importance that may be placed upon having at least one son. This may be because of the different male and female roles, with the male having a more dominant role in relation to the female. It may be significant as the family name and finances may only be passed to a male. The birth of a daughter may place strain upon the family finances if the tradition of providing a dowry on marriage is followed. Despite this, just because an individual belongs to a particular community, it cannot be assumed that they will automatically prefer a male baby over a female baby.

Naming the baby and naming systems

Some families do not allocate a name to the baby straight away. Many cultures name the baby on significant days according to particular traditions. For example, a male baby in the Jewish faith is traditionally named on the eighth day, which usually coincides with the day of circumcision.

In Sikhism the baby may not be named until the mother is well enough to go to the Gurdwara or temple, where the naming ceremony takes place. In Hinduism the baby's horoscope may be worked out from the exact time of birth by the pandit or holy man who may choose the first letter of the baby's name. The complete name may be chosen by an older member of the family (Schott and Henley, 1996).

There are many different naming systems throughout the world and most will not follow the pattern of the British system. It is imperative that the correct format of the name is recorded as the retrieval of results and records will rely upon this and if the name is recorded incorrectly it could lead to errors and confusion. The following examples are features that may be found in different naming systems (Schott and Henley, 1996):

- names which are exclusively male or female;
- the personal name may be placed first;

- the personal name may consist of two parts;
- some naming systems include a religious name which may or may not be used on its own;
- some systems may not have a shared family name;
- the family name may be placed first;
- a woman may not change her name on marriage, the husband's family name may be added to her own.

Examples of traditional naming systems can be found in the scenarios at the end of the chapter.

Feeding

Some communities follow the practice of not giving colostrum to the baby due to the belief that it may be unclean or have poor nutritional value. Even if colostrum is discarded and the baby given formula feed, lactation can still be established and breastfeeding can be successful (Sheikh and Gatrad, 2001). The cultural tradition of discarding colostrum may go against religious teachings which means that they are at odds. This means that the health education aspects of promoting breastfeeding need to be delivered in a culturally sensitive manner (Sheikh and Gatrad, 2001).

Privacy when breastfeeding may be extremely important and some women may be reluctant to breastfeed unless they have the guarantee of complete privacy in a side room. The need for privacy and maintaining modesty may be paramount and lead some women to delay initial attempts at breastfeeding until they are discharged home (Singh, 2007).

Settling the baby

It may be common practice in some Western societies to reduce the amount of handling newborn babies receive and, once settled, to leave them in the cot for long periods of time. In other societies it may be common for babies to be constantly in the mother's company; carried, cuddled and handled (Holland and Hogg, 2001).

Hygiene

In the Islamic faith the baby's head is shaved on the sixth or seventh day, as a symbol of removing the impurities of birth. It is common for Muslim boys and Jewish boys to be circumcised within approximately four weeks of birth and, in some cases, the procedure may be performed within the first few days of birth (Schott and Henley, 1996).

If the baby is wearing symbolic bracelets or symbolic threads care must be taken when dressing the baby or changing cot linen to make sure that the bracelets do not get thrown away. If the baby is in an incubator and cannot wear the bracelets it may be possible to place them inside the incubator near the baby.

People from a traditional Chinese culture may follow the belief of hot and cold and may fear that bathing the baby may result in the baby becoming overly chilled. This may also result in the baby being wrapped in several layers (Schott and Henley, 1996).

Prayer and religious observances

Many faiths require prayers to be said up to three times a day with additional prayers on significant days. In the Islamic faith prayers are said five times a day. In Sikhism prayers are performed early in the morning, at sunset and before going to bed. Ritual washing may need to take place before prayer.

In 2003 The Department of Health published a best practice guide to meet the religious and spiritual needs of clients and staff. One of the fundamental principles set out in the document is for the provision of suitable spaces for prayer and reflection. If parents want to pray it may be helpful to provide a private area, such as a side room with a hand basin and running water. Sometimes parents may prefer to pray at the cot side. If a prayer mat is needed, parents may be grateful for the offer of a clean sheet.

The parents may turn to religious leaders for help and healing and may want the religious leader present at discussions with health care practitioners. In Islam the Imam is a spiritual leader and parents may take great comfort from consulting him for guidance as well as prayer (Salas and Jadhav, 2004). Verses from the Quran may be written by the Imam for the parents to hold or place next to the baby.

Postnatal care

Some women may want to follow the traditional practice of staying at home or at their mother's home for up to 40 days following the birth, for rest and recuperation. This is common in many cultures including the traditional Chinese culture and traditional South Asian culture. During this time the baby is often cared for by female relatives and brought to the mother for breastfeeding. In order for the new mother to recuperate she may be washed by female relatives, given nutritious food and not expected to undertake domestic chores. Consequently women may find it unusual to be asked to care for themselves as well as the baby while in hospital. Trips to a baby or health clinic may be acceptable for some, but for others this may not be allowed and therefore the health care practitioner may need to visit the mother and baby at home.

It may not always be possible for women to undertake this period of rest or to have the support both physically and emotionally of females from their own community. Women may be separated from their extended family by thousands of miles or they may be the only female from a particular community living in an area. When women expect to follow this tradition but are unable to, they may become worried that their physical and mental health or the health of the baby may be affected (Sookhoo, 2003).

Visiting

Visiting a new baby or an ill baby and its family may be extremely important and an obligation that needs to be met by members of the extended family and friends, which may mean many people visiting at the same time. For example, this custom is common in the gypsy community with many travelling great distances to celebrate the birth or give support if the baby is ill (Jones, 2007).

Practices around dying and death

It must not be assumed that what may be common practices around the death of an adult will be practices that will accompany stillbirth or the death of a baby (Schott and Henley, 1996). Some families may wish to wash and prepare the baby's body themselves or they may want religious leaders to perform last offices. It may be disrespectful for a non-faith individual to perform last offices and touch the body (Schott and Henley, 1996). The relatives will also know if jewellery, sacred threads and other religious objects should or should not be removed from the body. Hindus may wish to use holy water from the Ganges. Muslims may wish to use water from the sacred city of Mecca (Sheikh and Gatrad, 2001).

In Jewish law 'a baby who has not lived for 30 days is not legally considered to be a fully viable human being', which means that some families may not follow the traditional mourning rituals. However, other families may choose to do so (Schott and Henley, 1996, p. 337).

Post-mortems may not be acceptable to some individuals. This may be because post-mortems are seen as disrespectful to the human body and may delay the funeral. It may be very important to some families that the body is intact with all organs returned before cremation or burial (Schott and Henley, 1996).

Language and communication

In a health care setting communication between the practitioner and parents can be affected by many factors such as a language barrier, the use of medical terminology and anxiety. For parents whose first language is English it may be difficult to understand the terminology used by health care practitioners, so for parents who have limited command of English it is even more difficult. If the baby is ill the parents will naturally be worried and stressed, which may further inhibit their ability to communicate in English. This may result in the parents feeling even more demoralised, isolated and unable to convey what they want for their baby (McAvoy *et al.*, 2006).

In order to provide individualised and comprehensive care for the baby it may be necessary to use a professional interpreter. Professional interpreters undergo training and clearly understand the boundaries of their role. Unlike an advocate they are trained to remain neutral. They will be trained to maintain confidentiality and, in the case of interpreting for the parents of a baby, they will respect the rights of the parents when making decisions about the child's care (Kai *et al.*, 2006).

The sad case of Victoria Climbié illustrates the need to use the services of a professional interpreter. Victoria was from Côte d'Ivoire and spoke French. She was unable to learn English and was not allowed to go to school. It appears that when she came to the attention of the social services she was not questioned through a professional interpreter but through the woman who was caring for her and who was responsible for her injuries (Kai *et al.*, 2006).

One approach to facilitate culturally sensitive communication

It is important not to make assumptions about care. The only way to find out what a woman/family wants for their baby is to talk with them. Every communication you have with parents is one step closer to building a trusting relationship, so it is vitally important that you do not inadvertently cause distress. McAvoy *et al.* (2006) give examples of how communication can be enhanced and the following principles are based upon their work.

- You need to assess how fluent the parents are in English, as you may need to involve a professional interpreter.

- Remember that parents may be stressed, especially if their baby is ill, and this can interfere with speaking English and the ability to understand and follow the simplest of instructions.
- Find out if the woman/family is familiar with the routines and procedures in your clinical area; this might be their first contact with a UK hospital.
- It may be helpful to think about what you are going to say and form an explanation and/or identify in your head the most important points that need to be conveyed before you sit down with the woman.
- It is the responsibility of the health professional to welcome parents and put them at ease with positive verbal and non-verbal messages.
- Pronounce names correctly.
- The conversation may take longer so allow extra time for explanations to be repeated and for confirmation that the woman/family have understood.
- Ask questions in different ways to establish the level of understanding.
- It may be necessary to simplify your English by not using technical medical jargon.
- Speak clearly and slowly, repeat phrases if necessary, summarise what you have said.
- Try to give instructions or explanations in a logical sequence, cover a topic and then move on to the next one.
- It may be necessary to use pictures.
- Pay attention to your non-verbal language.
- When people become highly emotional they may revert to their first language, keep calm and accept this.
- Some families follow a hierarchical structure and it may be necessary to respect their wishes and include a senior family member/person in conversations.
- Give written information for parents to take away.

The following may be ways to open a conversation:

'I think it would help both of us if I knew what you expected from me (as a nurse/midwife) in relation to baby feeding/nappy changing/bathing...'

'Your baby will need feeding soon... what can I do to help you prepare for feeding?'

'I'd like to talk to you about the health benefits of colostrum/breast milk. Can you tell me how you feel about breastfeeding baby at birth because sometimes it's helpful to understand other people's explanations for things.'

'How do you feel about feeding your baby at birth?'

CONCLUSION

This chapter has discussed the need for health care practitioners to develop an awareness of the diversity that exists in the UK today. Culture, ethnicity, race and religion have been explored. As an introduction to the existence of difference and diversity of needs, some practices that exist around care of the baby have been presented. Due to the nature of diversity that exists in the UK today it is not possible for health care practitioners to know all the customs and traditions that apply to different groups. However, if practitioners do not make assumptions and understand the importance of asking the family what they want for their baby, family-centred and culturally sensitive care is more likely to be achieved.

Key points
- Health care professionals must be aware that ethnic and religious groups are not homogeneous and great diversity exists across and within groups. Generalisations about groups often lead to stereotypes.
- The traditions and customs that surround care of the baby will be adhered to by some and ignored by others.
- It is important to treat people as individuals.
- Do not make assumptions about people.

Exercises

1. Baby girl of Cheung Ng Wai-Yung
Mother: Cheung Ng Wai-Yung, 20 years old, from a traditional Chinese family.
Grandmother (Mother of Cheung Ng Wai-Yung): Cheung Mee-Tuan, born in Hong Kong and came to Britain in the 1960s.
Religion: Buddhism.
You are the health care professional caring for Cheung Ng Wai-Yung, who gave birth to a 3.5 kg baby girl at term. It is now four hours after the birth. The grandmother Mee-Tuan has wrapped the baby girl very tightly in two blankets, a hat and is now adding a sheepskin. The baby is red in the face, has wet hair and beads of sweat on her forehead, she is crying loudly. You begin to unwrap the baby girl. The grandmother, who does not speak English, begins to talk loudly in Cantonese. To lighten the situation you comment on how pretty and healthy the baby is. Granny and Wai-Yung exchange words in Cantonese and look very upset.
What explanations can you give for the reaction of Wai-Yung and the grandmother?

What cultural and/or religious information might you need in order to provide care that meets Wai-Yung's and the baby's needs?
What actions will you take?

2. Baby boy Mohammed Ra'uf
Mother: Fatma Bibi, 17 years old, born and educated in Bradford.
Father: Nasim Ahmed, born and educated in Bradford.
Grandfather (Fatma's father): Mohammed Al'tariq born in Pakistan and came to Britain in the 1970s.
Grandmother (Fatma's mother): Jamila Khatoon born in Pakistan and came to Britain in the 1980s.
Religion: Islam.
You are the health care practitioner caring for Fatma and her baby boy Mohammed Ra'uf. Fatma gave birth to a baby boy at 26 weeks' gestation. Unfortunately the unit where she delivered did not have available neonatal intensive care cots so she and baby were transferred to a unit 100 miles away. Her husband Nasim Ahmed is travelling to be with her; she is accompanied by her parents. Sadly Mohammed Ra'uf died.

Although you speak directly to Fatma she does not answer and her father does all the talking. You ask if a photograph should be taken of Mohammed Ra'uf. After a conversation in Punjabi the baby's grand-father declines, saying that it is not permitted on religious grounds. Your experience and intuition tell you that this may not be what Fatma wishes.

• What cultural and/or religious information might you need in order to provide care?
• What actions will you take?

3. What are the different ethnic groups in your local area?
Where would you go to find out information about the needs of people from these ethnic groups?
Identify the interpretation services used in the clinical area where you work.
Now you have read the chapter think of three ways the information will help you deliver culturally sensitive care.

REFERENCES

Bhopal, R. (2004) 'Glossary of terms relating to ethnicity and race: for reflection and debate'. *MIDIRS Midwifery Digest*, 14, (3); 413–418

Department of Health (2003) *NHS Chaplaincy: Meeting the religious and spiritual needs of patients and staff*. London: Department of Health

Department of Health (2004) *National Services Framework for Children, Young People and Maternity Services*. London: Department of Health

Helman, C. (2006) 'Forewords', in Papadopoulos, I. (ed) *Transcultural Health and Social Care Development of Culturally Competent Practitioners*. Edinburgh: Elsevier

Holland, K. and Hogg, C. (2001) *Cultural Awareness in Nursing and Healthcare*. London: Arnold

Jones, K. (2007) 'Midwives and travellers', in Richens, Y. (Ed.) *Challenges for Midwives volume 2: Current issues in midwifery series*. London: Quay Books Division

Kai, J., Briddon, D. and Beavan, J. (2006) 'Working with interpreters and advocates', in Kai, J. (Ed.) *Valuing diversity; A resource for health professionals training to respond to cultural diversity* (2nd Ed.). London: Royal College of General Practitioners

MacLachlan, M. (2006) *Culture and Health: A critical perspective towards global health* (2nd Ed.). Chichester: John Wiley

McAvoy, B., Spencer, J. and Kai, J. (2006) 'Enhancing communication', in Kai, J. (Ed.) *Valuing Diversity: A resource for health professionals training to respond to cultural diversity* (2nd Ed.). London: Royal College of General Practitioners

Nursing and Midwifery Council (2008) *The Code: Standards of conduct, performance and ethics for nurses and midwives*. London: Nursing and Midwifery Council

Office for National Statistics (2001) *Ethnicity and Religion from the April 2001 census*. Available at **www.statistics.gov.uk/CCI/nugget.asp?ID=764&Pos=4&ColRank=1&Rank=176** (accessed 27 January 2008)

Office for National Statistics (2007) *Population trends No. 130*. Available at **www.statistics.gov.uk/downloads/theme_population/Population_Trends_130_web.pdf** (accessed 27 January 08)

Salas, S. and Jadhav, S (2004) 'Meeting the needs of Muslim service users'. *Professional Nurse*, 20 (1): 22–24

Schott, J. and Henley, A. (1996) *Culture, Religion and Childbearing in a Multiracial Society*. London: Butterworth Heinemann

Sheikh, A. and Gatrad, A. (2001) 'Muslim birth practices'. *The Practising Midwife*, 4(4): 10–13

Singh, D. (2007) 'Supporting infant feeding in the Bangladeshi community', in Richens, Y. (Ed.) *Challenges for Midwives Volume 2: Current issues in midwifery series*. London: Quay Books Division

Sookhoo, D. (2003) ' "Race" and ethnicity', in Squire, C. (ed) *The Social Context of Birth*. Abingdon: Radcliffe Medical Press

Spencer, N. (2000) *Poverty and Child Health* (2nd Ed.). Abingdon: Radcliffe Medical Press

Useful Websites

The Multi Ethnic Learning and Teaching in Nursing (MELTING) project can be found at the website.

www.maryseacole.com/maryseacole/melting/validated.asp

Ethnicity and health specialist library **www.library.nhs.uk/ethnicity**

Chapter 10

Legal and Professional Issues
Amanda Williamson and Charlene Lobo

Chapter aims

To explore professional and legal issues in relation to nursing the neonate and to introduce the principles of child protection in practice.

Learning outcomes

By the end of this chapter you will be able to:

- discuss the legal principles that underpin health care practice;
- demonstrate an understanding of the professional and legal avenues that are available to hold a health care practitioner to account;
- discuss how a valid legal consent may be obtained;
- describe the rights of children in law;
- articulate the importance of child protection in relation to health care practice.

Mapping to standards of proficiency

Standards of Proficiency for Pre-registration Midwifery Education (SPME)
Examine and care for babies with specific health or social needs and refer to other professionals or agencies as appropriate. This will include:

- child protection

Practise in accordance with *The NMC Code of Professional Conduct: Standards for Conduct, Performance and Ethics* (NMC 2004), within the limitations of the individual's own competence, knowledge and sphere of professional practice, consistent with the legislation relating to midwifery practice.

Practise in accordance with relevant legislation. This will include:

- practising within the contemporary legal framework of midwifery

Standards of Proficiency for Pre-registration Nursing Education
Manage oneself, one's practice, and that of others, in accordance with the *NMC Code of Professional Conduct: Standards for Conduct, Performance and Ethics*, recognising one's own abilities and limitations.

Practise in accordance with an ethical and legal framework which ensures the primacy of patient and client interest and well-being and respects confidentiality.

NHS knowledge and skills framework (NHS KSF)
Core 4, Level 2
The worker:

a) discusses and agrees with the work team
   • the implications of direction, policies and strategies on their current practice.
f) constructively identifies issues with direction, policies and strategies in the interests of users and the public.

Core 5, level 2
The worker:

a) acts consistently with legislation, policies, procedures and other quality approaches and encourages others to do so.
b) works within the limits of own competence and levels of responsibility and accountability in the work team and organisation.
f) monitors the quality of work in own area and alerts others to quality issues.

INTRODUCTION

As a health care practitioner it is vital that you always work within your scope of practice and within the law. This chapter will explore key legal and professional issues that are integral to working as a health care practitioner.

CONFIDENTIALITY

Confidentiality is a key aspect of working as a health care professional and it is important that you respect the parents' and their baby's right to confidentiality. The NMC (2008) says that you must respect people's right to confidentiality and ensure that people are informed about how and why information is shared by those providing their care. The NMC (2008) goes on to say that you must disclose information if you believe that someone may be at risk of harm in line with the law of the country where you are practising. You have a duty to maintain confidentiality under particular Acts of Parliament; these include the Data Protection Act 1998 and the Human Rights Act 1998. Under the law of negligence (see below) you owe the patient confidentiality as part of your duty of care. Within your contract of employment you will also have a duty to maintain confidentiality. There are some areas in which there are exceptions to the duty of confidentiality. These may include statutory requirements such as notification of births and deaths, with the consent of the patient or a court order (Dimond, 2006).

ACCOUNTABILITY

Midwives and nurses who are registered with the Nursing and Midwifery Council (NMC) may be held accountable for their practice by their professional body, the Nursing and Midwifery Council, by the law or by their employer or, in some situations, by all three. Health care practitioners who are not registered with the NMC may be held to account for their actions by the law or by their employer. It is important that you always practise within your own capabilities and are always willing to say when you don't feel able to undertake a task that you have not been trained to undertake or do not feel competent to undertake.

The Nursing and Midwifery Council's function is to establish and improve standards of nursing and midwifery care in order to protect the public (NMC, 2007). The NMC will consider any allegations of professional misconduct and anyone may make a complaint to the NMC. In 2005–2006 1 378 allegations of misconduct were made to the NMC (NMC, 2006). These allegations are mainly made by employers (49 per cent), the police (19 per cent) and the public (22 per cent). Allegations may also be from supervisors of midwives, colleagues and the National Care Standards Commission or others. The NMC (2008) says that as a professional you are personally responsible for actions and omissions in your practice and must always be able to justify your decisions.

Murray and Zentner (1989, p. 88) state that accountability is 'being responsible for one's acts and being able to explain, define or measure in some way the results of decision making'. This definition makes it crucial that the health care practitioner accepts responsibility and is able to provide a sound rationale for their practice. The health care practitioner should also be able to demonstrate that the care given was safe and effective; this enables you to evaluate the outcomes of your care.

The Midwives Rules and Standards (2004) defines the scope of acceptable midwifery practice within law. It states that:

a practising midwife is responsible for providing midwifery care, in accordance with such standards as the Council may specify from time to time, to a woman and baby during the antenatal, intranatal and postnatal periods

(2004, p. 16)

If you adhere to *The Code: Standards of conduct, performance and ethics for nurses and midwives* (NMC, 2008) and/or *The Midwives Rules and Standards* (NMC, 2004) in your practice, it will help protect you from allegations of misconduct or litigation. It is therefore important when caring for mothers and their babies that the health care practitioner acts within their own scope of practice and within Trust guidelines wherever possible and seeks appropriate assistance. By doing this you are safeguarding your own practice as well as protecting the baby and their family.

Legal accountability

Health care practitioners are accountable in law for their actions and omissions. Depending upon the complaint made against them, legal proceedings may be initiated under criminal or civil law. The majority of medical cases initiated are generally civil (or tort). A tort concerns disputes between individuals. The state steps in as an intermediary to settle the dispute. The reasons that most proceedings are civil may well be the lower standard of proof required (i.e. on the balance of probabilities) and the possible payment of damages. In criminal law there is a higher standard of proof required (i.e. beyond reasonable doubt) and monetary reward in the form of criminal compensation is lower.

In order to prove a negligent action in civil (tort) law there are four criteria that must be met:

1. It must be proved that the professional owed the claimant a duty of care.
2. It must be proved that the duty of care was breached.
3. It must be proved that the harm was caused by the breach of the duty of care.
4. It must be proved that the harm was reasonably foreseeable as a result of that breach.

It is only when all four conditions have been proven that damages may be assessed and awarded.

DUTY OF CARE

Legally there is little doubt that a health care practitioner owes a duty of care to their clients. The definition of duty of care in law was established in

Donoghue v. *Stevenson* [1932] AC 562. At 580 it states: 'You must take reasonable care to avoid acts or omissions which you can reasonably foresee would be likely to injure your neighbour.' It goes on to say your neighbour is:

> ... persons who are so closely and directly affected by my act that I ought reasonably to have them in contemplation as being so affected when I am directing my mind to the acts or omissions which are called in question.

For the health care practitioner anyone they are caring for will be 'closely and directly' affected by their acts or omissions.

STANDARD OF CARE

The health care practitioner must practise to the standard of their peers. The test for the expected standard of care is known as the 'Bolam Test'. It is the principle applied to all professionals. It was first articulated in *Bolam* v. *Friern Hospital Management Committee* [1957] 2 All ER. 118 where, at 121, McNair, J. said:

> The test is the standard of the ordinary skilled man exercising and professing to have that special skill. A man need not possess the highest expert skill at the risk of being found negligent. It is well-established law that it is sufficient if he exercises the ordinary skill of an ordinary competent man exercising that particular art.

The courts will ascertain the standard of care, based upon accepted health care practice as it existed at the time. This means that you are judged according to the prevailing standard of your peers at the time the incident took place. This means if the incident occurred 12 years ago the standard would be the accepted practice at that time. The court may look to *The Code: Standards of conduct, performance and ethics for nurses and midwives* (NMC, 2008) and *The Midwives Rules and Standards* (NMC, 2004) prevailing at the time as well as other health care opinion to establish the accepted standard of care.

This emphasises the importance of practising to the agreed standard of national guidelines (such as the guidelines agreed by the National Institute for Health and Clinical Excellence), NHS Trust protocols and guidelines as well as guidelines from the NMC. Expert witnesses called by either legal side in a case may offer a professional opinion on whether or not the health care practitioner was working to acceptable standards of the day.

The current climate of fear of litigation within the NHS has led to a large number of regulations and guidelines being developed within individual Trusts. Hurwitz (2004) notes that guidelines do not actually set legal standards for clinical care, but they do provide the court with benchmarks by which to judge clinical decisions. Thus a health care professional must be able to justify any clinical decision they make in relation to a baby's care.

In delivering treatment *Bolam* is also the expected standard but not all medical mistakes are negligent. In *Whitehouse* v. *Jordan* [1981] 1 All ER 261 HL, the Master of the Rolls said:

> ... in a professional man, an error of judgement is not negligent. To test this I would suggest that you ask the average competent and careful practitioner: is this the sort of mistake that you yourself might have made? If he says 'yes even doing the best I could, it could have happened to me' then it is not negligent.

This means that the law affords some protection, in that you are required to work to the standard of your peers rather than to the level of an expert health care practitioner.

Causation

In order to prove causation a client must show that there was a causal link between the breach of care and the harm that occurred. That is to say, that the client must show that 'but for' the defendant's negligence the harm would not have occurred. In the case of *Wilsher* v. *Essex Area Health Authority* [1988] 1 All ER 871 it was held that the injury could have been attributable to a number of different agents. That meant that causation was not proven. This means that a health care practitioner may only be held responsible if it can be proven that their negligent action caused the harm. Therefore, even if a client making a complaint against a health care practitioner can prove there was a breach of the duty of care they must also prove that the harm was caused by the actions of the health care practitioner and that the harm was foreseeable at that time.

It is only when the four criteria have been proven – that the professional owed the claimant a duty of care and that the duty of care was breached; that the harm was caused by the breach of the duty of care and that the harm was reasonably foreseeable as a result of that breach – that damages will be assessed and awarded.

CRIMINAL LIABILITY

The health care practitioner may also be held to account under criminal law. Gross negligence on behalf of a professional leading to death may lead to a conviction for manslaughter. The test was established in *R* v. *Batemen* [1925)] 19 Cr App R 8. In this case it was stated that:

> the negligence of the accused went beyond a mere matter of compensation between subjects and showed such a disregard for the life and safety of others as to amount to a crime against the state and conduct deserving punishment.

The law has further been clarified in *R* v. *Adomako* [1995]1 AC 17. In this case the House of Lords held that the defendant was properly convicted of involuntary manslaughter if:

> the ordinary principles of the law of negligence apply to ascertain whether or not the defendant has been in breach of a duty of care towards the victim who has died. If such breach of duty is established the next question is whether that breach of duty caused the death of the victim. If so, the jury must go on to consider whether that breach of duty should be characterised as gross negligence and therefore as a crime.

It will be considered a crime if:

> having regard to the risk of death involved, the conduct of the defendant was so bad in all the circumstances as to amount in their [the jury's] judgement to a criminal act or omission.
>
> Lord Mackay at 178

Any health care practitioner who had been responsible for a baby and in which their actions may have led to the death of a baby could face criminal proceedings if they were found guilty of the test described above. A jury would need to find that they were guilty of gross negligence 'beyond reasonable doubt'. These cases are obviously extremely rare and any safe practitioner who practises within their code of conduct and rules and standards are very unlikely to find themselves in this situation.

Limitation

The Limitation Act 1980 allows that an action must be brought within three years of the infliction of the injury or from the time of knowledge of the injury. However, if the harm is to a fetus or neonate then the three-year period can start from the time they reach majority. Under section 11 and section 14 of the Act if a person is unaware of the injury or did not know negligence may have caused the injury, then the three-year period starts from the date they did or should have reasonably discovered the facts. Section 33 allows the court to overrule the three-year period. This means that it is vital that health care records pertaining to care in child-birth are kept in excess of 21 years. This means that a health care practitioner may still be called to account for cases in which they were involved a long time ago. Therefore good record keeping is essential.

CONSENT

Legal consent for adults was defined in *Schloendorff* v. *Society of NY Hospital* 105 NE 92 (NY1914) as,

> every human being of adult years and sound mind has a right to determine what shall be done with his own body; and a surgeon who performs an operation without the person's consent commits an assault.

Obviously, obtaining consent for babies will be different as they are unable to consent to treatment themselves. Legally you need only gain consent from one person with parental responsibility. However, it is good practice to involve those close to the baby with the decision-making process (DH, 2001). It is important that you are familiar with who may have parental responsibility for a baby (as discussed above) so that you are able to obtain a valid consent.

For consent to be valid the parent (or person with parental responsibility) must be:

- competent – that is to say capable of making that decision;
- acting voluntarily (not under pressure from anyone);
- given enough information to enable them to make the decision.

(DH, 2001)

It is vital that the health care practitioner remembers to explain all risks and consequences to the parents so that the parents may make an informed choice. The DH (2001) guidance says that in order to make an informed decision parents need information about:

- both the benefits and the risks of the treatment;
- what the treatment involves;
- the implications of not going ahead with the proposed treatment;
- any alternative treatments available.

If the mother herself is under 16 she will only be able to give consent if she is 'Gillick Competent'. This means that 'A child may consent to treatment if she has sufficient maturity and understanding to understand fully what is proposed' (*Gillick* v. *West Norfolk and Wisbech AHA* [1985] 3 All ER 402). Any child who is considered to be 'Gillick Competent' 'can consent to' treatment. However, a competent child's 'refusal' of treatment can be 'overridden' by either the courts or by those who have parental authority using something called its 'inherent jurisdiction'.

If the parent's first language is not English you may need to consider the use of an interpreter to translate for you when gaining a valid consent.

If you provide care in an emergency the NMC (2008) says that you should be able to demonstrate that you have acted in the best interests of the person. It will be the health care practitioner's responsibility to ensure that a valid consent is obtained for all care and treatments.

CHILD LAW

Children have a number of rights under the United Nations Convention on the Rights of the Child (UNCRC) 1989 and the European Convention of Human Rights (UCHR) now incorporated into English law via the Human Rights Act (HRA) 1998. The fetus does not obtain rights in law until it has been born. The rights of a mother to determine her own autonomy cannot be overruled because she is pregnant, even if her own life or that of the fetus is at risk. This was established in *St George's Health Care NHS Trust* v. *S* [1998] 2 FLR 728 where it was stated:

> a pregnant woman was entitled, as an adult of sound mind, to refuse medical treatment, even if her own life and that of the unborn child depended upon such treatment.

United Nations Convention on the Rights of the Child

The UNCRC was adopted by the United Nations on 20 November 1989. The convention was adopted to recognise that 'in all countries of the world there are children living in exceptionally difficult conditions, and that such children need special consideration' (United Nations, 1989). By 2000 almost every country in the world had signed and agreed to be bound by the provisions of the convention. The United Kingdom ratified the UNCRC on 16 December 1991. The Convention applies to every human being under the age of 18 (unless the age of majority is lower) (Article 1). States must respect the rights of the child without discrimination, irrespective of the child's 'race, colour, sex, language, religion, political or other opinion, national, ethnic or social origin, property, disability, birth or other status' (Article 2). Other significant articles in relation to neonatal care include:

- In actions concerning children the 'best interests of the child shall be a primary consideration' (Article 3).
- States shall respect the responsibilities, rights and duties of parents (Article 5).
- States must recognise that 'every child has an inherent right to life' (Article 6).
- Children have the right to have their birth registered and the 'right to know and be cared for by his or her parents' (Article 7).
- No child should be deprived of his or her right of access to health care services (Article 24).

Although these rights are not binding in law they will be taken into account in a judgement made in relation to a child.

Human Rights Act (HRA) 1998

Other important legislation that gives children rights is the HRA 1998. Previously courts only had to have consideration for the European Convention on Human Rights (ECHR). Now the HRA means it is unlawful for public authorities to act in a way that is incompatible with the ECHR. Particular rights that may be significant in neonatal care are:

- Article 2, everyone's Right to Life shall be protected by law;
- Article 3, no one shall be subjected to torture or inhuman or degrading treatment or punishment;
- Article 8, the right to respect for private and family life;
- Article 14, prohibition of discrimination.

Children Act 1989 and Adoption and Children Act 2002

The Children Act 1989 and the Adoption and Children Act 2002 are significant legislation in relation to children. There are two main parts of the Children Act 1989:

- Private Law Orders; these control behaviour of individuals towards each other.
- Public Law Orders that are involved in society's intervention in the affairs of the family.

Information box 1

Principles of the Children Act 1989
- The welfare of the child is of paramount importance.
- Wherever possible, children should be brought up and cared for within their families.
- Children should be safe and protected effectively if they are in danger.
- There should be minimal delay in proceedings.
- Courts only to make an order if to do so is better than making no order at all.
- Children and parents to be kept informed of events.
- Parents continue to have responsibility for children even if the child is no longer living with them.

When making any decision in regard to a child the court will take account of the following welfare checklist (s 1(3)).

- Ascertainable wishes and feelings of the child concerned.
- Child's physical, emotional and educational needs.
- Likely effect on the child of any change in his or her circumstances.
- Age, sex, background.
- Any harm which the child suffered or is at risk of suffering.
- How capable parents or any other person in relation to the order are, in being able to meet the child's needs.

The Children Act 1989 also introduced the concept of Parental Responsibility. This is defined in Section 3 (1) as 'all the rights, duties, powers and responsibilities which by law a parent has in relation to the child and his property'. Who has Parental Responsibility?

- Mother – automatically.
- Father – automatically if the father's name is on the birth certificate (The Adoption and Children Act, 2002).
- If the father's name is not on the birth certificate he must apply for a court order to gain parental responsibility.
- Guardians by court order or by will, written appointment (s 5).
- Foster parents (s 12).
- Local Authority under a care order (s 33) or Emergency Protection Order (s 44).

The Children Act 1989 also introduced Section 8 orders. These are private law orders made in relation to the child and include Residence Orders, Contact Orders, Prohibited Steps Orders and Specific Issues Orders.

Public Law Orders

The Local Authority (LA) has a number of powers and duties towards children. It also has a number of responsibilities to provide services for children in 'need'. S 17(10) defines a child in need as:

1. The child is unlikely to achieve or maintain or have the opportunity of achieving or maintaining a reasonable standard of health or development without provisions of services.
2. The child's health or development is likely to be significantly impaired, or further impaired without the provision of such services.
3. The child is disabled.

The LA must provide a range of services appropriate to those children's needs and promote their welfare (s 17). The LA must investigate any claims that a child is at risk of 'significant harm' (s 31.(2) (a)). Significant harm is further defined in s 31(10): 'Where the question whether harm suffered by a child is significant turns on the child's health or development, his health or development shall be compared with that which could reasonably be expected of a similar child.'

Children Act 2004

The Children Act 2004 provides the legal underpinning for *Every Child Matters* (DH, 2004). The key points from this Act are as follows.

- That professionals working with children are required by law to co-operate with each other, to improve the 'well-being' of children. 'Well-being' is the term used to define the five *Every Child Matters* outcomes:
  1. be healthy;
  2. stay safe;
  3. enjoy and achieve;
  4. make a positive contribution;
  5. achieve economic well-being.

- There should be an electronic file on every child where there are concerns about their welfare.
- There should be a director of Children's Services in each council and Statutory Local Safeguarding Children Boards.
- Under the Act new powers for central government were given to enable them to intervene if children's social services fall below minimum standards.

SAFEGUARDING CHILDREN – ISSUES FOR PRACTICE

Although the law sets quite clear guidelines for the practice of safeguarding children, within the context of busy hospital wards/clinical practice the competing priorities of different professionals and the difficulty for practitioners in establishing evidence (especially for emotional vulnerability) means that safeguarding children becomes quite a complex issue for nurses and midwives in practice.

Defining child maltreatment is challenging and can be interpreted in many different ways. Child abuse is a dynamic socially constructed phenomenon. This means that what society regards as causing harm to children has changed over time and has different meanings in different cultures. For example, we see this within the United Kingdom where smacking children has in the past been regarded as an accepted form of chastisement but is now very controversial. In Scotland unacceptable levels of physical punishment are prohibited under the law but this is not so in England.

Definitions of abuse and neglect are linked to society's views on what is acceptable or unacceptable. For example, the current focus on the importance of the maternal–infant relationship to healthy emotional and psychosocial development of children may be regarded as 'ethnocentric'. This means that as practitioners we need to be mindful that the prevailing European view of the 'mother's role' or the 'family' does not negatively influence the judgements we make on child vulnerability. For example, Munro (2007) claims that those views on child-rearing where attachment is to the primary caregiver in the context of the nuclear family disregards other child-rearing practices where the extended family and father's roles might be equally significant. This cultural and contextual positioning of 'good enough' parenting is difficult to determine and can create uncertainty and anxiety for practitioners (Powell, 2007). 'Good enough parenting satisfies the health, safety and developmental needs' of the child (NCIPCA, 1996).

In the light of these varying positions it is important to understand that any decisions about protecting children should never be carried out independently and should always be discussed with and made in consultation with other members of the team or named professionals for safeguarding children.

In practice making decisions on whether a child's needs are related to parental abuse or neglect and whether they are experiencing harm or at risk of experiencing significant harm are very complex. Professionals are faced with high criticism from the media and public when they err in their decision-making process in assessing the child as a victim of abuse, or in misjudging the severity of the danger that they are in, and this helps to contribute to defensive practice (Munro, 2007). That leads to a focus of risk assessment rather than supportive interventions.

Decisions often have to be made with limited knowledge and consequently the judgements and decisions on interventions tend to contain a degree of uncertainty. Professionals have to sift through the information, interpret its significance and make difficult judgements and decisions.

Munro (2007) describes decision-making as being based on analytical and intuitive reasoning; analytical reasoning is formal, explicit and logical, intuition is based on unconscious processes. This can be quite problematic for practitioners. Firstly, in terms of analytical reasoning, the acute clinical environment not only makes it difficult to support the mother–infant relationship but the environment also makes it difficult to identify or evidence any dysfunctionality in the care-giving behaviours. Secondly, in terms of intuitive reasoning, we need to be aware that our own emotional states can be aroused by particular care-giving states and this can impact and influence the judgements we make in relation to assessment. Clinical supervision therefore becomes imperative in the delivery of good-quality care within the context of safeguarding children.

Another dilemma in practice is that practitioners find it very hard to move between mindsets of support and suspicion. Practitioners are often faced with the paradox of adopting a primary supportive stance in care delivery on the one hand, at the same time being mindful that infants and particularly preterm infants are very vulnerable to harm. Corby (2006) raises questions about the correlation between preterm infants and child abuse, arguing that too much of a focus is put on the bonding relationship and less consideration is taken of the social factors that contribute to the stress experienced by such families. Again, ensuring good clinical supervision in practice is vital to safe good-quality practice.

In conclusion, if you suspect that a baby is at risk of harm, you should follow the underpinning principles which are:

- be aware and follow your local policies and procedures;
- always discuss your concerns with someone else;
- refer on to the appropriate person or agency;
- always follow up referrals.

Key points
- Confidentiality is a key part of working as a health care practitioner.
- You may be held to account for your actions professionally and legally.
- You should always work within the scope of your practice and never undertake a task that you feel unsure of or that you have not been trained to undertake.
- You should be aware of children's rights when caring for babies.
- You should always obtain a valid consent before commencing care for a baby.

Exercises

1. You are working on the postnatal ward that is really busy. The midwife in charge asks you to perform a neonatal screening test; however, you haven't covered this in your training yet. What should you do and why?
2. You are asked to take the temperature of a newly born baby. What should you ask the parents before taking the baby's temperature and why?

REFERENCES

Adoption and Children Act 2002

Bolam v. *Friern Hospital Management Committee* [1957] 2 All ER 118

Children Act 1989

Children Act 2004

Corby, B. (2006) *Child abuse* (3rd Ed.). Berkshire: McGraw-Hill

Data Protection Act 1998

Department of Health (2001) *Seeking consent: working with children.* London: Department of Health

Department of Health (2004) *Every Child Matters*. London: Department of Health

Dimond, B. (2006) *Legal Aspects of Midwifery* (3rd Ed.). Books for Midwives. Butterworth Heinemann Elsevier

Donoghue v. Stevenson [1932] AC 562

Gillick v. *West Norfolk and Wisbech AHA* [1985] 3 All ER 402

Hurwitz, B. (2004) 'How does evidence based guidance influence determinations of medical negligence?' *British Medical Journal*, 329: 1024–1028

Human Rights Act 1998

Limitation Act 1980

Maynard v. *West Midlands Regional Health Authority* [1985] 1 All ER 635

Munro, E. (2007) *Child Protection*. London: Sage

Murray, B.R. and Zentner, J.P. (1989) (adapted by C. Howells) *Nursing Concepts for Health Promotion*. Englewood Cliffs, NJ: Prentice Hall

National Commission of Inquiry into the Prevention of Child Abuse (NCIPCA) (1996) *Childhood Matters*, Vol. 1. London: HMSO

Nursing and Midwifery Council (2004) *Midwives Rules and Standards*. London: NMC

Nursing and Midwifery Council (2004) *The NMC Code of Professional Conduct: Standards for conduct, performance and ethics*. London: NMC

Nursing and Midwifery Council (2006) *Fitness to Practise Annual Report*. London: NMC

NMC (2007) What the NMC does at **www.nmc-uk.org/(hrpre0vkuis cuu45g145afaq)/aArticle.aspx?ArticleID=25**

Nursing and Midwifery Council (2008) *The Code: Standard of conduct, performance and ethics for nurses and midwives*. London: NMC

Powell, C. (2007) *Safeguarding Children and Young People: a Guide for Nurses and Midwives*. Berkshire: McGraw-Hill

Re W (a minor) medical treatment [1992] 4 All ER 627

R v. *Adomako* [1995]1 AC 17

R v. *Batemen* [1925] 19 Cr App R 8.

Schloendorff v. *Society of NY Hospital* 105 NE 92 (NY1914)

Sidaway v. *Bethlem RHG* [1985] 1 All ER 643

St George's Health Care NHS Trust v. *S* [1998] 2 FLR 728

United Nations Convention on the Rights of the Child 1989

Whitehouse v. *Jordan* [1981] 1 All ER 261 HL

Wilsher v. *Essex Area Health Authority* [1988] 1 All ER 871

Appendix: Organisations and Roles in Neonatal Care

British Medical Association (BMA)
www.bma.org.uk
The British Medical Association is the doctors' professional organisation, representing doctors in the UK, looking after the professional and personal needs of their members.

British Association of Perinatal Medicine (BAPM)
www.bapm.org
A multidisciplinary association that provides advice and services to improve the standards of perinatal care in the British Isles.

Confidential Enquiry into Maternal and Child Health (CEMACH)
www.cemach.org.uk
This organisation aims to improve the health of mothers, babies and children by carrying out confidential enquiries on a nationwide basis. They publish the findings and make recommendations to improve care.

Department of Health (DH)
www.dh.gov.uk
A Government department that aims to improve the health and well-being of people in England.

The Foundation for the Study of Infant Deaths (FSID)
www.fsid.org.uk
The Foundation is a UK charity aiming to prevent unexpected deaths in infancy and promote infant health.

General Practitioner (GP)
Royal College of General Practitioners
www.rcgp.org.uk
A doctor who provides primary care in the community.

Health care assistant
Health care assistants work within hospital or community settings under the guidance of a qualified health care professional.

Midwife
Royal College of Midwives
www.rcm.org.uk
A midwife provides advice, care and support for women, their partners and families during the preconceptual, antenatal, intranatal and postnatal periods.

National Health Service (NHS)
www.nhs.uk
The NHS is a publicly funded body which provides a comprehensive range of services throughout primary and community health care, intermediate care and hospital-based care. Services also include health promotion, disease prevention, self-care, rehabilitation and aftercare.

National Institute for Health and Clinical Excellence (NICE)
www.nice.org.uk
NICE is an independent organisation responsible for providing national guidance on promoting good health and preventing and treating ill health.

National Screening Committee (NSC)
www.nsc.nhs.uk
The UK National Screening Committee (NSC) advises ministers, the devolved national assemblies and the Scottish Parliament on all aspects of screening policy.

National Service Frameworks (NSF)
www.dh.gov.uk
National Service Frameworks (NSFs) are long term strategies for improving specific areas of care. They set national standards, identify key interventions and put in place agreed time scales for implementation.

Neonatalologist
A doctor who specialises in care of the newborn.

Neonatal Nurse

National Association of Neonatal Nurses

www.nann.org

A nurse who specialises in the care of premature and sick babies.

Nurse

Royal College of Nursing

www.rcn.org.uk

A nurse works as part of a multidisciplinary team caring for people's health and well-being in hospital or community.

Nursery nurses

Nursery nurses and nursery assistants provide care for children up to five years of age, in hospitals and in the community.

Nursing and Midwifery Council (NMC)

www.nmc-uk.org

The Nursing and Midwifery Council (NMC) safeguards the health and well-being of the public by continually regulating, reviewing and promoting nursing and midwifery standards.

Paediatrician

The Royal College of Paediatrics and Child Health.

www.rcpch.ac.uk

Paediatricians are qualified doctors who specialise in the diagnosis and treatment of disease and the care of children.

Index